ESCAPING HASHIMOTO

REVERSING HYPOTHYROIDISM AND GRAVES' DISEASE

I0414067

By IRVIN SYMONETTE

DISCLAIMER

The material provided in this book is not intended to be a medical guide in any form. Neither is it to be considered an in-depth study of the immune system. It is not meant to replace or substitute professional medical advice. As a victim of Hashimoto thyroiditis, I only want to share my experience and reasoning for the different treatments and therapies that I adopted on my way to recovering my health.

The material is for informational purposes only. Whatever recommendations are provided is not intended to diagnose, treat, or cure any disease. The statements provided have not been assessed by any health, food, or drug administration. If you see something of interest to you and would like to integrate it into your treatment, make sure to do so under the supervision of a qualified medical professional.

Contents

THE SURPRISE

It was supposed to be just another regular check-up. I had lost a little edge in life and a permanent lethargic feeling had settled in over me. My memory had also been a little dull, but I thought it was nothing to be concerned about. After all, I wasn't twenty-five anymore, and age brings changes.

A couple of days after the doctor's visit, my phone rang. At the other end of the line was a concerned voice; it was the doctor. After seeing the results of my blood tests, he wanted to see me in his office first thing the following morning.

Once I was in the doctor's office, he told me, "Your blood test reveals that you have a thyroid problem which needs immediate attention. Your thyroid-stimulating hormone count is at 187. The normal range is between 0 and 3.5. In all my years of practicing medicine, I have never seen readings as high as this.

"These numbers indicate that your pituitary glands are desperately trying to get your thyroid gland working, but it isn't responding. Your thyroid gland has virtually stopped working. I find it hard to believe that you still have the energy to be walking around. Nevertheless, here you are in front of me. You're in danger of passing out at any moment, and we must take emergency measures starting immediately."

He wrote a prescription and instructed me to, "Take one as soon as you reach home and one every day after that, preferably at the same time daily. In the meantime, we will conduct a few more tests to determine the extent of the damage."

After another round of blood tests, an ultrasound, and an X-ray, the verdict was in: "You have Hashimoto thyroiditis."

I'd never so much as heard of an illness by that name. But at least it wasn't cancer, so I was relieved.

"Your body is committing suicide," the doctor explained. "Your immune system attacks the thyroid gland and has destroyed it. Unfortunately, the disease is in the advanced stages and there is nothing that we can do about it. The cause of this illness is unknown, and there is currently no cure. If we even had a cure, the damage inflicted upon the thyroid gland is beyond repair; it is virtually dead. There's no possibility that it will ever return to normal function again. Your T4 count is only two while the normal range is between twelve and twenty-two."

Here I was with an incurable disease and a thyroid gland that had been irreversibly damaged. Now that was unfortunate!

The specialist was quick to offer his support by saying: "It isn't all doom and gloom. The medication that I've prescribed for you will allow you to continue living a normal life with virtually no side effects. You won't even notice that your thyroid is not functioning anymore.

"As a matter of fact, we have people who've had their thyroid removed surgically and by taking this medication, they've been able to go on with their lives without losing a beat."

As we left the doctor's office, I commented to my wife, "Maybe cancer would've been a better diagnosis."

There are rumors everywhere that cancer can be cured by natural means, but for this Hashimoto disease, it seemed that I am going to need two miracles: one, to stop the disease, and the other to rebuild my thyroid gland.

Naturally, this required a second opinion. The next doctor wondered, "How are you even capable of walking into my office? In your condition that shouldn't be possible."

It was now time for a third opinion.

"According to these numbers, you shouldn't even be alive. You're living on borrowed time, my friend. You could go into a coma any day now and possibly die."

Forget that comment—let's go for a fourth opinion.

"You are the worst case of this illness I have ever encountered in Canada." By this time, my TSH level had gone "off the chart," according to the doctor. Which meant that the TSH level was higher than the machine was programmed to register. "Only in Africa have I seen people this far gone. By the way, where are you from?"

Funny doctor! A fifth opinion shouldn't hurt, right?

"In my forty years of practicing medicine, I have never seen anybody recover from this disease—especially not anyone as far gone as you are."

So, I said to my wife, "I've had enough of the doctors' opinions. I am too young for you to attend my funeral. You may marry again and have me rolling in my grave. We can't have that happening, so it's time to work on a plan to postpone it."

I was resisting the idea of swallowing the little pill called Synthroid that the doctor had prescribed to me. I thought that the negative diagnoses they were giving me were to convince me that I really had no other choices.

As time went by, I became convinced that these doctors were right. That reversing the sickness was a fight against death. The odds were stacked against us.

I then turned my attention to alternative remedies. After a couple of liver-detoxifying treatments and a few herb supplements, nothing changed. My health continued its downward spiral. Another natural health practitioner promised that in one year's time, I would be as good as new. But at the end of twelve months, there was no improvement. I even had to quit my job, unable to work by that time.

Another health practitioner commented on my condition, saying, "Piece of cake." But that cake was never baked.

Conventional doctors and those who practice healing using alternative means seemed to agree on one thing: the source of this condition is unknown. There is no known cure. This disease could only be managed. Some natural health practitioners admit that in cases of Hashimoto thyroiditis, they make an exception and recommend that levothyroxine be taken along with natural remedies.

Information about this illness is so limited that anyone would believe that Hashimoto thyroiditis is a new disease. When you do a web search, Google will return millions of results, but most of the information is repetitive and offers very little value to the understanding of Hashimoto. And yet Synthroid and levothyroxine, the medications that are often prescribed for this condition, are the most prescribed medications, by the number of monthly prescriptions, both in Canada and the US (WebMD 2015 most-prescribed-top-selling-drugs, Commonly Prescribed Medications, 2015).

I've learned one thing in confronting Hashimoto thyroiditis; one cannot rely entirely on a health practitioner. The only thing that everybody seems to know about this illness is that they don't know anything about it. You cannot treat an illness that you don't understand!

There is a good chance that you're reading this book because you've been on the same merry-go-round as me. In this hit-and-miss game, it seems the misses have overwhelmingly prevailed. For this reason, I endeavored to acquire as much knowledge as I could about this disease.

By medical standards, Hashimoto thyroiditis is incurable. With this understanding, I started out on my six-year journey through the valley of the shadow of death. (Hashimoto thyroiditis 2015).

We live in a scientific age. We rely on scientific minds to provide us with answers and guidance. For many of us, if the scientific community doesn't confirm it, then it isn't real. Fortunately for us, science has provided all the evidence that we need to understand Hashimoto thyroiditis.

I had no idea how long it was going to take me to recover. This journey had the appearance of a dead-end road right from the start. There is nothing easy about this condition. Every day you wake up, the struggle begins all over again. You really don't have the luxury of making long-term plans, as all you can do is take one day at a time.

In the following pages, I will share with you the knowledge that allowed me to break free from Hashimoto thyroiditis. What do you say? Can we start our journey?

UNDERSTANDING HASHIMOTO

The only effective way to confront Hashimoto thyroiditis is by acquiring a comprehensive understanding of the disease. It will not take long before you realize that the doctors are right in their claim to know little—if anything at all—about this autoimmune condition. You are almost on your own.

If you remember, though, ignorance is what brought us to this stage of the illness. We were not aware that there was a fire burning inside of us, and now that we do, it's time to put it out.

So, as we embark on this adventure with high hopes of recovery, knowledge will prove to be indispensable. The better we understand this illness, the higher our chances of breaking the shackles it has on us. Knowledge will give us the advantage as we work in close partnership with our health professionals.

The human body's basic functioning and structural biological components are cells. Cells are the smallest unit of life, the building blocks. We are made up of trillions of cells, divided into over 200 different types. Together, they form the best performing machine in the world. All the functions of our body take place on a cellular level. Sickness and well-being both depend on the condition of the cells that makes up our body. To understand a disease, we must first understand how these cells work.

Cells have guidelines for normal behavior. These guidelines are coded messages commonly known as genes. A normal cell never deviates from the rules contained in its genes. A cell, at times, may lose a number of vital control systems when the DNA becomes modified, damaged, or lost. We then become sick.

Illness is the direct consequence of deviating from these genetic guidelines. We may do this presumptuously, or by ignorance, but it does not make a difference. The result of cell degeneration is the same: disease.

Illness could be brought on by environmental, chemical, nutritional, emotional, or spiritual factors, which could pose quite a challenge when trying to find out what has caused a modification in a cell's behavior.

In an article entitled "pH of the Human Body Is Critical for Health," Gary Tunsky, a world-renowned cellular disease specialist, declared that: "A healthy body is determined by the health of each of its single cells. All disease originates at a cellular level and not at the organ or system level. Healthy cells create healthy tissues. Healthy tissues create healthy organs like the heart and lungs. Healthy organs create healthy systems like the endocrine system or the immune system. And health systems make up a healthy body."

A diseased body is a clear indication that the cells have become dysfunctional. A cell's job consists of protecting, healing, repairing, and regenerating. Failure to perform any of these tasks is a sign that the cell is sick.

Since the good health of our cells is the key to our overall health, how do we maintain healthy cells?

The condition we have come to know as "sickness" is usually the result of our own creation. Sickness is not something that comes upon us overnight or by chance. Neither is it a matter of having bad luck or misfortune. We manufacture it moment by moment, one bite at a time and often, one thought at a time.

A few people have brought sickness on themselves by willfully breaking the laws of good health, but for most of us, following the highway of ignorance got us here. We do not know what, how, where, or when we deviated from the path of healthy living. We simply believed that we would be healthy forever until we found ourselves blindsided by sickness. However, the fact remains that our sickness is of our own doing.

The cells of the body are very resilient. If they once worked properly, they could be persuaded to do so again. With a determined effort, the right knowledge, and a capable health care professional, we could coax our cells back to a state where they can live up to their design, doing what cells do: providing us with good health.

Months and even years may go by before a cell changes its behavior. Thus, getting an abnormal cell to work properly again is a process that will not happen overnight.

THE IMMUNE SYSTEM

Hashimoto thyroiditis is a disease of the immune system. So, let us take some time to acquaint ourselves with it.

The immune system is made up of an elaborate network of specialized cells, tissues, and organs. It is a complex defense mechanism of biological processes and structures that are designed to detect and neutralize a wide variety of invaders such as viruses, parasites, and bacteria. It relies on the dynamic and effective communication abilities among all the cells in the system to recognize and respond to alien substances called *antigens*. An antigen is anything capable of inducing an immune system reaction.

All living organisms, including unicellular ones such as bacteria, have an immune system. However, many mammals (including humans) have a much more advanced immune system. It possesses an immunological memory which keeps a record of all the pathogens (a disease-causing micro-organism) that it has encountered so that it can react faster in any subsequent confrontation.

When we have sufficient biological defenses to avoid infections and diseases, we call that a state of immunity. This is the body's ability to resist and prevent any harmful microbe from entering the body. If the immune system is working well, we would never become sick, but if even one component becomes damaged or inactive, we easily become victims of many maladies.

The immune system is composed of many independent cell types with specialized functions. They engulf bacteria, kill parasites or tumor-producing cells, and destroy viral-infected cells. Even though this process may include many substances, organs and—in the end—the entire body, it is essentially a one-to-one battle between cells. So, when we talk about the immune system, we are talking about cells.

Some of the cells of the immune system are T cells, B cells, natural killer (NK) cells, leukocytes, macrophages, and granulocytes. The organs of the immune system are the bone marrow, the thymus, the spleen, and the lymph nodes. The bone marrow is not an organ itself, but in discussions about the immune system, it is usually grouped among the other organs that either produce cells or substances that enable the immune system to perform effectively in keeping us disease-free.

A malfunction of the immune system occurs when something goes wrong within the DNA of each cell, changing its prime directive. This malfunction falls under one of three categories: immune deficiency, hypersensitivity, or autoimmunity.

Immune deficiency occurs when the immune system's ability to defend the body against any given pathogen is diminished. In some cases, this is mainly due to aging. However, other factors such as obesity, alcoholism, and drug use are active contributors to poor immune system function.

Malnutrition is the most common reason for immune deficiency. Another cause is losing the thymus by mutation or surgical removal. Immune deficiency could also be inherited or acquired as in the case of AIDS.

Hypersensitivity is an undesirable overreaction of the immune system in response to certain chemicals considered being non-threatening. This immune system reaction is commonly known as *allergies* or *intolerance*. Some symptoms of this condition are eye irritation, rash, nasal congestion, nausea, and vomiting.

There are four classifications of hypersensitivity based on the length of time it takes for symptoms to appear. Type 1 hypersensitivity produces an immediate reaction. Types 2, 3, and 4 hypersensitivities could take days to develop, and their reactions range from mild discomforts to death.

Autoimmunity is an organism's abnormal immune system response against its own tissues and organs. The immune system loses its identifying ability to the point that it becomes incapable of distinguishing between a pathogen and the cells of one's own body. Because of this dysfunction, the immune system targets organs and tissues of our body and systematically destroys them.

Hashimoto is considered an autoimmune disease, yet to date, the manner of development of Hashimoto thyroiditis is still not fully comprehended (Gryalska, Matyjaszek-Matuszek, Pysik, and Rolinski 2015).

AUTOIMMUNITY

Within the last thirty years, the field of clinical immunology has been subject to some paradoxes that contradict the positions adopted by most physicians. The puzzle of autoimmunity is an example of this. (Poletaev 2014)

The classical definition of autoimmunity is: "The system of immune responses of an organism against its own healthy cells and tissues. Any disease that results from such an aberrant immune response is termed an autoimmune disease (Wikipedia 2016)."

When considering self-directed tissue inflammation, there are major difficulties with this concept of autoimmunity. Healthy, living cells within our body have a set of proteins on their outer membrane. They are essentially ID tags for our cells. This is how our immune system recognizes our own cells versus foreign bodies (Study.com 2016). If this ID is intact, the body's cells do not come under attack. In many tentatively labeled autoimmune diseases, the cells do not lose their identity. A gradual appreciation of these facts has led to the revision of the definition of autoimmunity (McDermott and McGonagle 2006; Wikipedia 2016).

Despite the predominant ideas about the built-in aggressive nature of the immune system, autoimmunity is a permanently present phenomenon in every individual, which does not always reflect the potentially self-destructive nature of the immune system (Poletaev 2014).

The idea that the immune system functions by making a distinction between self and non-self has also come under scrutiny for failing to explain a number of findings (McDermott and McGonagle 2006). For example, why do we fail to reject tumors, even when many clearly express new or mutated proteins? Why do most of us harbor autoreactive lymphocytes without any sign of autoimmune disease while a few individuals will succumb to them?

Almost 120 years ago, Ilya Ilyich Metchnikoff, a Russian zoologist best known for his pioneering research in immunology, suggested that the main purpose of the immune system is not a "struggle" against invading pathogens.

The fight of the immune system's cells against outside agent, is just one of the facets of a much wider biological purpose of the immune system, which is responsible for the control of dynamic self-maintenance, self-repairing, self-construction, self-optimization, and perpetual self-harmonization of an organism in spite of the imperfections of the body and pressure from the environment (Agapov et al. 2012).

It is evident that autoimmunity is not a disease, but a necessity. The immune system is directly involved in the physiological activities of the body. Therefore, its functions are directed rather inward, not outward, and are based on the intrinsic recognizing components of itself or self-tolerance. (Poletaev 2014).

According to GenScript, a biotech company specializing in biological research and drug discovery/development services, self-tolerance is "the ability of the immune system to recognize self-produced antigens as a non-threat, while appropriate mounting a response to foreign substances. This balance of immunological defense and self-tolerance is critical for normal physiological function and overall health."

Quintana and Howard (2006) describe the immune system as a two-edged sword. "It recognizes and destroys non-self-targets, protecting us against environmental pathogens. Sometimes it aims at self-targets, causing autoimmune disease. Lately, however, we have become aware of the beneficial role of autoimmunity in some biological processes such as tissue repair."

Autoimmunity is the natural resistance with which a person is born. It provides resistances through several physical, chemical, and cellular approaches (Wikipedia 2016).

Autoimmunity occurs during pregnancy, in which certain antibodies are passed from the maternal blood into the fetal bloodstream in the form of IgG antibodies (McDermott and McGonagle 2006). A normal immune system makes antibodies that recognize and prevent foreign organisms from causing infection. They are produced by plasma cells in response to an antigen.

Antibodies that are formed in response to elements of one's own body are called autoantibodies. Autoantibodies themselves are harmless, but in large amounts, they can suggest the presence of an autoimmune disease. Sometimes they bind to immune cells like mast cells and basophils. This binding activates these cells to perform functions such as secretion of inflammatory chemicals (McDermott and McGonagle 2006).

Antibodies that are directed toward self (for example, thyroid antibodies) are called *natural autoantibodies* and are part of a physiological mechanism for cleansing the organism of its own catabolic products. Meanwhile, classical antibodies serve to clear the body of foreign invading agents.

The realization in the past two decades that autoantibodies reacting with various self-antigens are common in normal animals and humans has led to intensive research on the origin and the physiologic role of these "natural autoantibodies" (Shoenfeld and Tomer 1988; Casali and Elkon 2008). These natural autoantibodies are detectable in the serum of healthy individuals before deliberate immunization. In contrast, regular immune antibodies are produced in response to the introduction of antigens to the immune system.

Zouali (2015) says that natural autoantibodies are "frequently directed to intracellular structures, rather than to cell-surface antigens." In a variety of experimental models, they have been found to play a role in protection against infectious agents and maintaining balance in the internal environment of the body.

Mahla (2015) describes natural antibodies as functionally not restricted to protect the host from invading pathogens, although they are a key regulator of waste management in the system, generated through cell disintegration. In the case of autoimmune disease, proper functioning of the immune system machinery could be hampered either by hyper-responses or by tissue degeneration, causing the natural antibodies to operate unrestricted.

Natural autoimmunity is an inborn process that occurs normally in the body. Natural autoantibodies and autoreactive cells are found in healthy subjects, and they are directed to a specific and limited set of self-molecules (John Hopkins Autoimmune Disease Research Center 2016).

Autoimmunity is not a disease, but a normal function of the immune system (American Autoimmune Related Diseases Association, Inc. 2016). However, constant or excessive activation of the natural autoimmune mechanism could result in autoimmune disease (MedicineNet.com 2016; MedlinePlus 2016).

One of the factors that contribute to autoimmune disease is the decrease in population of T cells, cells that maintain natural immunity. As the number of T cells declines, so does tolerance to self-antigens (Asano et al. 1996). The autoimmune disease then results from a hyperactive immune system (Microbiology and Immunology On-line 2016).

The concept of autoimmunity upon which this book is based is that *autoimmunity is the natural resistance with which a person is born, usually referred to as natural immunity or self-tolerance* (Wikipedia 2016).

Autoimmunity is normal, not a disease.

Hashimoto

Autoimmune disorders occur when the immune system cells go out of control and begin to destroy healthy organs and tissues in the body instead of protecting them. In the case of Hashimoto thyroiditis, healthy thyroid tissues become inflamed, resulting in the destruction of thyroid cells and ultimately hypothyroidism. The disease is named after the Japanese specialist, Hakaru Hashimoto, who first described it in 1912.

There are many autoimmune disorders, and Hashimoto thyroiditis stands at the top of the list. Other autoimmune disorders are rheumatoid arthritis, diabetes Mellitus type 1, systemic lupus, and Graves' disease (McCoy 2015).

Hashimoto thyroiditis is the most prevalent form of inflammation of the thyroid gland, and the most common thyroid disorder in America (Milas 2016). It affects people of all ages, including children, but is more predominant in middle-aged women (Mayo Clinic Staff 2014).

We develop Hashimoto thyroiditis when the immune system becomes hyperactive, making too many autoantibodies—a sign of inflammation. This, however, is no indication that the autoantibodies are defective. An autoimmune disease is the result of the constant activation of natural immunity. This condition may be caused by some deficiencies in the immune system (Agapov et al.

2012; Grammatikos and Tsokos 2012; eLS 2015; Mahle 2015; Shoenfeld and Tomer 1988).

Hashimoto is a slow-developing disease which takes years before its effects could be seen or felt. By the time we become aware of its presence, the disease is in its later stages and is difficult to treat, much less reverse.

In the initial stages, Hashimoto usually produces symptoms that are very mild and easily overlooked, or are misdiagnosed as hyperthyroidism. This is because in the early stages, when the thyroid gland is undergoing the ill effects of inflammation, the cells begin to disintegrate and there is blood leakage. This blood is loaded with thyroid hormones, which are then converted into energy. We experience a spike in energy, which could be interpreted as hyperthyroidism. However, this could be so mild that it may go unnoticed. As the sickness advances though, the thyroid gland will become weaker and our energy level decreases.

Some health care professionals remain baffled by this autoimmune disorder. Just finding someone knowledgeable about Hashimoto disease is like looking for a needle in a haystack.

According to the conventional medical and scientific community, there is no known cure for Hashimoto thyroiditis. This means that there is no available medication to accomplish that purpose. The disease is simply allowed to run its course of systematic destruction of the thyroid gland (MedicineNet.com 2016).

Though science has not yet provided us with a cure, if we pay attention to the results of the numerous studies conducted, we would discover that with natural medicine, Hashimoto *is* curable.

Thyroiditis

The term *thyroiditis* refers to the inflammation of the thyroid gland. The classic sign of an autoimmune disease is inflammation. It is the body's attempt at self-protection, the aim being to remove harmful stimuli, damaged cells, irritants, or pathogens and begin the healing process (American Thyroid Association 2016; Nordqvist 2015).

They are two types of inflammation that affect the thyroid gland: acute inflammation, which lasts only a few months, and chronic inflammation.

The immune system cells involved in acute inflammation are basophils, eosinophils, and neutrophils. They secrete inflammatory substances like histamine, peroxidase, heparin, and chondroitin sulfate. These inflammatory chemicals can destroy normal cells and dissolving connective tissues (Weiss 1989).

For surrounding tissue not to be damaged by inflammatory chemicals, the inflammation must be terminated. This failure will result in chronic inflammation and cellular destruction (Abbas and Kumar 1999; Manzoor 2012) known as *bystander tissue damage* (Wikipedia 2016; Nordqvist 2015; MedicineNet.com 2016).

When acute inflammation is activated too often, it becomes chronic. Chronic inflammation is mediated by macrophages, dendritic cells, histiocytes, Kupffer cells, and mast cells (Alm 1983; Wikipedia 2016).

Chronic inflammation is characterized by the dominating presence of macrophage in the injured tissue. These cells are powerful defensive agents of the body. The toxins they release (including reactive oxygen species) are injurious to the organism's own tissues, as well as invading agents. Consequently, chronic inflammation is almost always accompanied by tissue destruction (Gardner et al. 2011; Elenkov 2004; Allison et al. 1978; Heikenwälder 2016; Laskin and Pendino 1995).

One fascinating aspect of a macrophage is its ability to know which cells to destroy and which ones to leave alone (Study.com 2016).

Over a century ago, Ilya Ilyich Metchnikoff described how phagocytic cells, rather than antibodies, are responsible for inflammatory tissue reactions against foreign antigens. Today we know it's true (McDermott and McGonagle 2006).

There are many forms of thyroid inflammation, and each receives its name based on what causes it:

- **Postpartum or silent thyroiditis** makes its appearance after a woman has given birth. It is thought to be the result of necessary changes that occur in the immune system during pregnancy (Wikipedia 2016).

- **Subacute thyroiditis** is a rare condition thought to be caused by a viral infection. It often occurs after a viral infection of the ears, sinus, and throat, such as mumps, the flu, or a cold (MedlinePlus 2016).

- **Drug-induced thyroiditis** is brought on by medications such as amiodarone, lithium, and interferon (American Academy of Family Physicians 2014).

- **Radiation-induced thyroiditis** results from radioactive therapy to treat hyperthyroidism, or from radiation to treat head and neck cancer or lymphoma (Alterio et al. 2004).

- **Acute thyroiditis** is an infectious thyroiditis known also as suppurative thyroiditis, microbial inflammatory thyroiditis, pyrogenic thyroiditis, and bacterial thyroiditis. It is an infection most often caused by bacteria, but can also be attributed to a fungal or parasitic infection in an immunocompromised host (John Lazarus, MA, MD, FRCP, FRCOG, FACE; Dr. James Hennessey, M.D.).

- **Riedel thyroiditis**, a rare inflammatory process involving the thyroid and surrounding cervical tissue, is associated with various forms of systemic fibrosis (Hennessey 2011).

Most of these types of inflammations lead to hypothyroidism and are easily treated. But in combination with other factors (such as allergy, stress, nutritional deficiency, toxins, or adrenal fatigue), any of them can be contributing factors to Hashimoto thyroiditis.

Hashimoto is a complex condition involving many components, but there is one key point that you should keep in mind as we journey toward recovery: Hashimoto is an inflammatory disease.

Putting out the fire of inflammation has to be our number one task.

Under Attack

With Hashimoto thyroiditis, the term "*attack*" is often mentioned. How should it be understood? What constitutes an "attack" on the thyroid gland?

An attack is defined as:

- To act violently against (someone or something);
- To try to hurt, injure, or destroy (something or someone);
- To criticize (someone or something) in a very harsh and severe way;
- To begin to work on or deal with (something, such as a problem) in a determined and eager way.

These definitions do not represent the attitude of the immune system against the thyroid gland.

The first response of the immune system against most intruders is the release of adrenaline or a similar chemical that produces inflammation. If these chemicals are secreted in or around the thyroid gland regularly, at some point, it will become inflamed. The inflammation process is considered an attack.

The current school of thought with regards to Hashimoto is that the immune system is reacting against elements of the thyroid. There are no invaders involved. The immune system thinks that the thyroid gland itself is the enemy, and even worse than that, the thyroid gland is what is causing these attacks. However, there has been no evidence, scientific or otherwise, to support the concept of this suicidal attitude of the immune system toward the thyroid gland (Boskey and Wint 2012).

These attacks on the thyroid gland are provoked by a third party, and they are usually on and off. They may last for one to three hours at a time, can happen multiple times during the day, and extend on for weeks, months, or years depending on the triggering agent.

The times when the thyroid gland is not under attack could last for a few hours, or it could go for weeks and up to six months. However, the most likely scenario is that these attacks will become more intense and regular as we age, and our health deteriorates.

So, if you were to be treated for this disease and six months go by without any attacks, the thyroid gland may begin to recover and resume normal production of the thyroid hormone. This happened to me and I mistakenly interpreted this little break as an indication that the disease was in remission. Then the thyroiditis flared up again and, three years later, I was still struggling to improve.

When the thyroid gland is chronically inflamed, it may remain stable for periods of time. However, there are certain elements that act as agents to make the inflammation flare up again. The most common triggers that we need to be aware of are bacteria, viruses, adrenaline, histamines, cortisol, gluten, and even pregnancy.

If you can successfully manage these triggers, the attacks will die down. With no attacks, there will be no thyroiditis of any sort, not even Hashimoto thyroiditis.

Remove the trigger and you eliminate the attacks.

Hashimoto thyroiditis is a slow yet steady destroyer. It will not relent until the thyroid gland is completely disabled. Even if you are taking Synthroid and you are capable of resuming a somewhat normal life, you are still vulnerable to other autoimmune disorders and many undesirable symptoms such as infertility, miscarriages, birth defects, high cholesterol, heart failure, seizures, stroke, coma, type 1 diabetes, multiple sclerosis, Addison's disease, chronic fatigue syndrome, fibromyalgia, pernicious anemia, and premature death (Roddick 2015; American Autoimmune Related Diseases Association, Inc. 2016).

Hashimoto thyroiditis follows this progression:

- First, there is an intruding pathogen.

- Second, in response to this intruder, the immune system produces inflammation-causing chemicals.

- Third, this chronic inflammation causes the cells of the thyroid gland to disintegrate.

- Fourth, in response to this disintegration, the immune system produces autoantibodies that target the thyroid gland and its proteins.

- Fifth, the result is an underactive thyroid.

So, if we successfully eliminate the inflammation, the Hashimoto thyroiditis empire falls, and everything else, like a domino effect, will be taken care of.

Any release of inflammation-causing chemicals, in or around the thyroid gland, constitutes an "attack" on the gland.

Hypothyroidism

Before moving on, let us familiarize ourselves with hypothyroidism. The thyroid gland consists of two connected lobes forming a butterfly-shaped gland located in the front of the neck, just beneath Adam's apple. One of its functions is to control how quickly the body utilizes energy. It manufactures thyroid hormones and controls the body's sensitivity to other hormones.

The thyroid gland is also responsible for regulating the growth and function of other systems in our body. Without these thyroid hormones, there would be no life.

When the thyroid gland does not produce enough hormones, it can make you feel fatigued, tired, and weak. This condition is known as *hypothyroidism* (Norman 2016).

There are many disorders that can affect the thyroid gland. Among those are thyroid nodules, thyroid tumors and cancer, thyroiditis, hyperthyroidism, and hypothyroidism. Our focus here is on the latter which is the result of Hashimoto thyroiditis.

The early signs of hypothyroidism are: increased sensitivity to cold, constipation, low heart rate, fatigue, weight gain, decreased sweating, muscle cramps, joint pain, dry and itchy skin, thin and brittle fingernails, rapid thoughts, depression, poor muscle tone, infertility, menstrual cycle problems, and elevated cholesterol levels. Later symptoms are goiters, slow speech, a hoarse, breaking voice, low body temperature, dry and puffy skin, mood swings, stress, acute fatigue syndrome, hypotension, and carpal tunnel syndrome (MedlinePlus 2016).

Some advanced symptoms are hair loss, impaired memory, impaired cognitive function, sluggish reflexes, increased need for sleep, decreased libido in men, and decreased sense of smell and taste.

No one will suffer from all of these symptoms, but if you have Hashimoto, you will exhibit most of them.

There are many books, articles, blogs, and health practitioners that could shed insight on recovering from hypothyroidism. However, if this condition was caused by Hashimoto thyroiditis, it's an entirely different story. With

Hashimoto, we are not dealing with just a sick, underactive gland, but with a damaged, mutilated thyroid, which presents its own challenges.

To complicate things even more, with Hashimoto thyroiditis, the hypothyroidism is not just caused by damaged cells, but also by the presence of thyroid-stimulating hormone (TSH) blocking antibodies. TSH-blocking antibodies attach themselves to the receptors on the thyroid gland normally reserved for thyroid stimulating hormones. This maneuver prevents the thyroid from being stimulated, so there is no production of thyroid hormones. If these autoantibodies were to be removed, the hypothyroid condition would disappear. This is much easier than it sounds.

According to experts, damages to the thyroid gland can be so extensive, to the point that any recovery is considered impossible (New York Times 2016).

Do not be alarmed by the statements in the previous paragraph. That is just a professional opinion. Scientific evidence confirms, that once the autoimmune attack ends, the damaged thyroid can generate new cells (Dr. Izabeella Wents farm D.2016l)

Hashimoto is reversible!

CONCEPTS AND MISCONCEPTIONS

Hashimoto thyroiditis is the most common autoimmune condition, yet it also is one of the most misunderstood (Boskey and Wint 2012; MedlinePlus 2015). Herein lies the problem, how can anyone treat a disease which they do not understand?

The scientific community has not been able to produce an alternative remedy for Hashimoto superior to the one that they already have, which is Synthroid because they are looking for something that could be patented. However, we have been provided with the results of so many studies and research that we should not have any problem using this information in our fight against Hashimoto thyroiditis. Unfortunately, although this information is out there, it is not being used by many of those who believe in alternative medicine.

An internet search will provide you with millions of results about Hashimoto, but mostly theories and conflicting opinions. This gives us a flawed concept of Hashimoto thyroiditis.

If you are unaware of what to look for, any attempts to explore this disease will reward you with a pile of nothing. Our ignorance is more damaging to us than the disease itself. We are lost in a jungle of recycled myths and fables offered to us by those who want to be heard but have nothing to say. Others hope that we would forget all about it and just swallow the pill.

Some of these theories make for good fairy tales but sound more like alternative nonsense. On the surface, everything looks and sounds rational, but dig a little deeper, and disappointment is all you will find.

Join me as we explore some of these misconceptions of Hashimoto thyroiditis.

Synthroid is the Only Solution

Conventional medicine's answer to Hashimoto thyroiditis is Synthroid, or one of its many cousins such as Levothyroxine or Eltroxin, which is a synthetic replacement for the thyroid hormone. This medication becomes a life sentence as it must be taken daily for the remainder of one's life. It has few minor side effects, but it allows one to resume a somewhat normal life.

Synthroid helps to eliminate the symptoms of Hashimoto but does nothing to halt the advance of the disease. This thyroid hormone synthetic replacement will abandon you to the whims of the disease, and why not? After all, the disease is incurable, isn't that right?

I don't think so!

Some people report that Synthroid *does not* work for them. In my opinion, there are four reasons that could render this drug ineffective:

- Synthroid is a man-made replacement, which is chemically similar, but essentially different from the real thyroid hormone. With some people, the body simply does not recognize the medication and targets it for destruction. Don't be surprised if Levothyroxine does nothing for you. It may keep us alive for a while, but if you want to have vibrant health, do not count on it. Synthetic thyroid hormone is equivalent to being on a life support system.

- The body could be missing the deiodinase enzyme group necessary to convert T4 into T3. So, it doesn't really matter if the T4 is the body's own creation or man-made, it would still have no effect on our system (Nordqvist 2015).

- When we consume wheat, even if we don't have celiac disease, gluten can block the thyroid hormone from entering the cells. Whether it's real thyroid hormones or a synthetic replacement, any access to the cells is denied (Paleo Leap 2016).

- High levels of cortisol cause thyroid hormone resistance in the cells, like what happens with insulin resistance, which makes it difficult for the cells to absorb Synthroid (Virginia Hopkins Test Kits 2016).

Some health professionals recommend taking prescription medicine while following a natural treatment protocol at the same time.

Those who advocate this approach do so base on two premises:

- First, that the disease is not curable;
- Second, damages done to the thyroid gland are irreversible.

I tried this approach at the insistence of my doctor. It is like attempting to cross a busy intersection blindfolded, unaware of the dangers that may come your way.

Synthroid, in eliminating the symptoms associated with Hashimoto, provides a sense of well-being, while there is the ongoing destruction of the thyroid gland by the disease.

The immune system creates TSH-blocking autoantibodies in response to excess thyroid hormones T4 in the blood. The excess hormone resulting from taking the medication will induce the immune system to shut the thyroid gland down by way of producing more thyrotropin receptor autoantibodies. So, any treatment to improve the functioning of the thyroid gland would be useless because it would have already been neutralized by the medication.

This means that taking the tablet could turn out to be counterproductive, and could even eliminate your chances of full recovery. If you are not a very health-conscious individual or are not disciplined enough to stick to a plan, Synthroid is a good solution.

We know that we are sick because of the way we feel, our body communicates with us, and this is also true if the body is recovering from an illness. If we hope at all to overcome this disease, we need to understand the language that the body speaks. It is a matter of becoming aware of how the body responds to everything, whether it is food, therapies, or supplements. All the body's responses need to be accurately interpreted.

Synthroid eliminates that advantage because it will make the body feel somewhat normal, overriding the symptoms of the disease that are eating away at it. To better treat the body, at some point, Synthroid will have to be eliminated or the dose greatly reduced, otherwise, it will lengthen or prevent recovery.

My main problem with this so-called solution is that one may appear to be normal, yet inside our body, a fire is burning in the form of Hashimoto thyroiditis. Worst of all, there is no guarantee that when the thyroid gland is annihilated, the disease will be over. It may well continue to eat away at other systems and organs of the body.

This illness, if not treated, could progress and develop into other autoimmune conditions, such as:

- Vitiligo: a disease that destroys the cell that gives color to your skin.

- Rheumatoid arthritis: a disease that affects the lining of the joints throughout the body.

- Addison's disease: an illness that affects the adrenal glands, which helps the body to respond to stress and regulates blood pressure, water, and salt balance.

- Type 1 diabetes: a disease that causes the blood sugar level to be too high.

- Pernicious anemia: a disease that keeps your body from absorbing B_{12} and making enough healthy blood cells.

- Lupus: a disease that can damage many parts of the body, like the joints, skin, blood vessels, and other organs.

We may end up taking more medication to hide the symptoms, but Hashimoto will eventually catch up and get the best of us. We then end our days as victims of medication.

This doesn't sound promising, right? Go and visit a senior home. Notice that they are all alive, but are sedated with medication to hide their myriads of symptoms. A lot of these people should not be there, but unrestrained diseases have destroyed vital organs and systems in their bodies, and so they are alive, but barely living.

I have no desire to become like them. Personally, I would prefer to live a shorter life than live a long life with a body riddled with disease, so I took the option to go against popular opinion and seek a cure by natural means.

My personal point of view is that health professionals with the opinion that the medication should be taken along with alternative medicine is a clear indication that they are not knowledgeable enough to be of much help in reversing Hashimoto thyroiditis.

When you understand the dynamics of Hashimoto for yourself, you will realize that the medication is not essential. If you have the conviction that you must take the medication, always under dose. In doing so, you will ensure that the thyroid will not be completely neutralized. You will still recover, but it will take a little longer.

A Weak Immune System

One school of thought promotes the idea that Hashimoto thyroiditis is the result of a weak immune system, because as they say, only a weak immune system would attack the body. So, the natural approach is to strengthen the system.

Can you believe that the driving force behind such an aggressive disease as Hashimoto thyroiditis is a weak immune system? The very notion is contradictory! If the immune system was weak, then we wouldn't have an autoimmune illness, but an immunodeficiency disease. Why? Because for the immune system to be weak, it must be lacking in something. In other words, it is *deficient*.

Consider another point: just imagine that you are in a fight, and you are at the losing end of the struggle. Would you give your antagonist an energy drink before the fight is over, or would you want to sedate him?

I was recommended to strengthen the immune system. Wrong idea—it resulted in even more damage done to the thyroid gland.

Hashimoto thyroiditis is a disease in which the immune system is hyperactive, manufacturing anti-thyroid antibodies in abundance. The last time I checked, hyperactivity was not a characteristic of weakness. As a matter of fact, with Hashimoto thyroiditis, a debilitated immune system would be a plus, because you don't want a strong immune system attacking your thyroid gland. Then again, a weak immune system would not can do so much damage to the gland.

Here is another point to consider: the health of the immune system is determined by the number of white blood cells, and a low white blood cell count is never a problem in Hashimoto because that count is always high— very high. A weak immune system and low white blood cell count go hand in hand, not the other way around.

In fairness to the theory of a weakened immune system, in Hashimoto thyroiditis, the system may be sometimes out of balance, meaning one arm of the immune system is weak while the other is strong. However, this condition occurs only when the system becomes suppressed.

Hashimoto thyroiditis is not the result of a weak immune system. The T_h1 arm of the immune system may be suppressed thanks to chemicals like cortisol, but remember, suppression is not the same as weakness. Furthermore, it is counterproductive to attempt to balance or strengthen the system while the gland is still inflamed, because then the fire will increase, more damage will be inflicted on the gland, and your condition will deteriorate.

If your initial approach to this disease is to strengthen the immune system, you will inevitably run into many regrettable consequences because you will be strengthening the very cells that are inflaming the gland.

Current scientific evidence suggests that autoimmune diseases are caused not by a weak immune system, but by a strong one (Callier 2016).

It is not about a strong or a weak immune system, but balance. Instead of making efforts to strengthen the immune system, we should consider balancing it. Even so, the immune system could only be balanced after the inflammation is under control.

The System is Suicidal

Autoantibodies are specialized in recognizing molecules, bearing in mind that all regulatory processes in an organism are based upon complementary intermolecular recognition.

We have, in existence, a specific network of autoantibodies that recognizes resident or self-antigens. The old school of thought considers autoimmune disease as one in which the body initiates an immune response against its own healthy tissues, mistaking them for harmful pathogens or irritants. The body produces antibodies that attack these tissues, leading to deterioration and, in some cases, their destruction (Wikipedia 2016).

In the last few years, researchers have noticed that many chronic inflammatory human disorders do not fit the criteria of autoimmune disease. They have established that tissue inflammation against self is not necessarily caused by abnormal T and B cells (McDermott and McGonagle 2006). They are in the process of changing the criteria for the classification of autoimmune diseases. Hashimoto thyroiditis is one of those diseases that may be affected by the new classification.

Even though autoantibodies are used to determine the presence of Hashimoto, researchers have not been able to directly link them to the destruction of the thyroid gland (Gaberšček and Zaletel 2011). Despite the high prevalence of Hashimoto thyroiditis, the exact mechanisms responsible for its development are still not completely understood (Chistiakov 2005).

In the past, autoimmunity was the result of a defect or abnormality with the immune system. Now, autoimmunity is regarded as a harmless, normal process of the immune system. Making antibodies that act against its own tissues is normal, and the immune system never loses the ability to distinguish between self and non-self (John Hopkins Autoimmune Disease Research Center 2016; Agapov et al. 2012).

On the internet, you will find many Hashimoto theories that have no scientific support. The classification of these attacks as self-provoked is one example. We know that there is a trigger, but we are led to believe that our body is the trigger; it is provoking itself.

However, there is a fire starter lurking somewhere.

Given the proper circumstances, any inflammation of the thyroid gland could progress into Hashimoto thyroiditis. How is that so?

Let us assume that the thyroid gland becomes a victim of a viral invasion. The immune system responds by releasing an inflammatory chemical like histamine, causing the thyroid to become inflamed. If the initial response of the immune system is strong enough to neutralize this pathogen, the attack would be called off and the inflammation will disappear, meaning a quick recovery!

Suppose now that the virus influx is overwhelming to the point that it becomes chronic. The immune system finds itself in a constant confrontation, continually sending histamine to the thyroid gland, so the inflammation becomes chronic. Because of this ever-present inflammation, the cells of the thyroid gland are weakened and begin to disintegrate. Thyroid hormones, along with thyroglobulin and thyroid peroxidase, leak into the bloodstream. The thyroid hormone causes an increase in energy and speeds up metabolism on a whole, looking pretty much like an overactive thyroid or hyperthyroidism.

With thyroglobulin and thyroid peroxidase running wild, the purity of the blood is now compromised, so the immune system goes into action again and produces autoantibodies against those two substances to clear them from the bloodstream. However, the work of the immune system is not over. It also produces TSH-blocking antibodies to reduce the production of thyroid hormones. Now we have full-blown Hashimoto thyroiditis.

If you followed our illustration closely, the only thing abnormal about this sequence of events is that they were all chronic. It started with a consistent battle against a virus, leading to the release of pro-inflammatory chemicals by the immune system, which then gave way to the disintegration of the thyroid gland. This, in turn, caused the production of antibodies that ultimately resulted in hypothyroidism.

Free yourself of the chronic viral infusion, and you free yourself of histamine, the inflammation, the damaged gland, the immune response, the autoantibodies, and, in the end, Hashimoto thyroiditis.

This example was meant to highlight one point: the inflammation has a *cause*. The immune system was being hyper-stimulated. It was constantly being spurred on by a viral infection.

Autoimmune diseases are classified and recognized by the presence of autoantibodies. We sometimes misinterpret that information to mean that the antibodies are causing the inflammation, but scientific evidence does not corroborate that misconception.

Hashimoto is an autoimmune disorder. However, it does not really meet the criteria to be considered as such, since there are no antibodies or immune system responses against any of the actual cells of the thyroid gland (McDermott and McGonagle 2006). The autoantibodies are directed against the elements of one's own body, but those autoantibodies are not causing any damage to the thyroid gland, and no part of the thyroid gland is provoking the immune system into action. The thyroid gland here is a victim, not necessarily of the immune system, but, of the inflammation.

We misinterpret the presence of autoantibodies as evidence of provocation, but this is not the case. The production of autoantibodies is the immune system's effort to protect and heal the ailing gland.

Consider one more example. Let us liken the immune system to a perfectly functioning door, one that opens and closes without problems. Now we take a door-jam and put it under the door in the open position. The door cannot be closed unless we remove the door stopper. If we placed the door stopper under the door while it was closed, we would be unable to open it unless we removed the stopper. The stopper here represents the T helper cells.

Nothing is wrong with the immune system, but we must find and eliminate the cause of what is interfering with the immune system mechanism.

Some experts tell us that most Hashimoto cases are caused by infections. That may be subject to discussion because there are many other causes (Trentini 2015; Desailloud and Hober 2009; Babal et al. 2015). The thyroid gland is not damaged because the immune system attacks it directly. When the immune system responds to an antigen, the inflammatory chemicals secreted by dendritic and macrophage cell against the intruder damage the cells of the thyroid gland. This is known as bystander damage (Chistiakov 2005).

The immune system does not directly, attack

the thyroid gland.

Defective Antibodies

Another misconception is that the immune system malfunctions, and, as a result, manufacture defective antibodies. Most people run along with this myth, but it is misleading. Please hear me out.

The main function of the immune system is to maintain the body in perfect health. This is achieved by mounting attacks against anything that could disrupt health and cause disease. Nevertheless, it also has many more attributes, most of them unexplored.

Recent advances in B cell biology have capitalized on old findings and demonstrated that B cells also release a broad variety of cytokines, "small proteins released by cells that have a specific effect on the interactions between cells, on communications between cells, or on the behavior of cells" (MedicineNet.com 2016).

A functional B cell subset, regulatory B cells (Bregs), "has recently been shown to contribute to the maintenance of the fine equilibrium required for tolerance. Bregs restrains the excessive inflammatory responses that occur during autoimmune diseases, or that can be caused by unresolved infections" (Bosma and Mauri 2012).

Antibodies are produced by B plasma cells in response to an antigen and they function in many ways:

- They bind directly to pathogens, preventing them from entering or damaging healthy cells;

- Stimulate other cells of the body to perform certain functions (Novimmune 2016);

- Can mark pathogens so that they can be identified and neutralized by other immune system cells (Novimmune 2016);

- According to researchers, antibodies are also effective in treating and reducing symptoms associated with inflammation (Baba et al. 1978; Holecek 2010; Dohi et al. 2009). Antithyroid antibodies, a part of the immune system, and are anti-inflammatory;

- Are not damaging to the organism and have protective properties (Grönwall et al. 2012; Shoenfeld and Toubi 2005);

- And are useful for clearing away dying cells and other debris. High levels of antibodies are also connected with longevity (Callier 2016).

Keep in mind that autoimmunity is not a disease, but a normal function of the immune system. This means that the autoantibodies are a part of a normal process of the immune system. This is called *low-level autoimmunity* or *natural immunity*. Autoimmunity is present in everyone and is harmless (John Hopkins Autoimmune Disease Research Center 2016).

For discussion, we could divide antibodies into two main groups:

- Natural antibodies, known as autoantibodies, are directed toward self-antigen (elements of one's own body). They are key regulators of body waste management, generated through cell disintegration in the system (Mahla 2015).

- Classical antibodies or regular antibodies, which serve to clear the body of foreign invading agents (Shoenfeld and Tomer 1988).

It's like a country that has two armed forces. The army takes care of foreign invaders, but when a citizen becomes a renegade, the police step in. Natural autoantibodies are like the police force while regular antibodies are equivalent to the armed forces of the body.

Natural autoantibodies are essential antibodies of the immunoglobulin M (IgM) Isotype, present in the circulation of normal humans and other mammalian species. They are detectable in the serum of healthy individuals. On the other hand, classic or regular antibodies are produced in response to the introduction of antigens to the immune system.

Natural autoantibodies are frequently directed to intracellular structures rather than to cell-surface antigens. They are harmless but suggest the presence of an autoimmune disease (Zouali 2015; Immune Deficiency Foundation, USA 2016).

The overproduction of natural autoantibodies will result in autoimmune diseases, such as Hashimoto thyroiditis. However, these natural autoantibodies never lose the ability to distinguish between self and non-self. So, the theory of loss of self-recognition resulting in the production of defective B cells, making defective antibodies is erroneous (Agapov et al. 2012; Grammatikos and Tsokos 2012; Mahla 2015; Shoenfeld and Tomer 1988).

The reference ranges for antithyroid antibodies (Elhomsy 2014) are as follows:

- Thyroid peroxidase antibody (TPOAb): Less than 35 IU/ml

- Thyroglobulin antibody (TgAb): Less than 20 IU/ml

- Thyroid-stimulating immunoglobulin antibody (TSI): Less than 140 percent of basal activity

- Thyroid-stimulating hormone (TSH) receptor binding inhibitor immunoglobulin (TBII) /TRAb: 1.75 IU/L or less

There is a range at which the level of these autoantibodies is considered normal. If they are normal, then the abnormality is not in the antibody itself, but in their quantity.

The anti-thyroid autoantibodies may cause damage by complement activation (Bès et al. 2002). This is to say that they do not do the damage themselves, they are only an accessory to the crime (Wikipedia 2016). Furthermore, there is absolutely no scientific evidence that directly links autoantibodies to the systematic destruction of the thyroid gland, neither by inflammation nor any other way (Djurica and Trbojević 2005).

It is well established in the scientific community that tissue inflammation against self, in this case, the thyroid gland, is not the result of abnormal B or T cells (McDermott and McGonagle 2006). There is no link connecting T cells with the inflammation, and neither is there any evidence that B cells cause it.

Targeting autoantibodies as defective is equivalent to taking an innocent suspect into custody. Our concern should be finding the cause of the immune system's over-activity.

Thyroid autoantibodies are normal, produced by a normal immune system.

Antibodies Destroy the Thyroid

There are three main thyroid autoantibodies identified:

- Thyroglobulin autoantibodies
- Antithyroid peroxidase autoantibodies
- Thyrotropin receptor autoantibodies

Thyroglobulin is a protein, and thyroid peroxidase an enzyme. They are part of the thyroid gland and are used to manufacture the thyroid hormone. Thyrotropin receptors respond to thyroid-stimulating hormones (Wikipedia 2016).

When the gland becomes damaged by inflammation, thyroid peroxidase and thyroglobulin leak into the blood where they do not belong, so the immune system finds it necessary to clear them from the bloodstream. It accomplishes this by sending out thyroid peroxidase and thyroglobulin antibodies to get the job done.

Thyroid peroxidase (TPO) and thyroglobulin autoantibodies have nothing to do with the destruction of the thyroid gland. There are some people that test positive for TPO antibodies but do not have thyroid disease, and there are others who may never test positive for any of these two autoantibodies and still have Hashimoto thyroiditis (Nippoldt 2015; American Association for Clinical Chemistry 2016). This is an indication that the presence of these autoantibodies in the blood is not conclusive evidence that one has Hashimoto thyroiditis.

Some health professionals have embraced the idea that the destruction of the thyroid gland is caused by thyroid peroxidase and thyroglobulin antibodies. However, these antibodies are not inflammatory, so how could they produce inflammation? What's more, according to Kids health (2015), antibodies are not capable of destroying anything on their own.

*Destruction of the thyroid gland
is not caused by thyroid autoantibodies.*

Other health care providers claim that the destruction of thyroid peroxidase and thyroglobulin contributes to the deterioration of the thyroid gland. However, it is worth noting that although these proteins are produced by the thyroid, they are not cells of the said gland. So, even *if* the immune system was to destroy all the thyroid peroxidase and thyroglobulins from the blood, it would have no adverse effects whatsoever on the cells of the thyroid gland itself. The thyroid would remain intact.

We should not be too concerned about thyroid peroxidase and thyroglobulin autoantibodies. Once the inflammation disappears and the thyroid gland heals, these antibodies will return to normal levels. Hashimoto thyroiditis is a T cell–mediated disease, meaning that the inflammation has T cells as arbitrators, not antibodies (Metcalfe et al. 2010; Chistiakov 2005).

Regulating Autoantibodies

Thyrotropin-receptor blocking autoantibodies, also known as thyroid-stimulating hormone (TSH) blocking antibodies and thyroid-stimulating autoantibodies, are a little more problematic.

In autoimmune diseases, there are usually two waves of antibody production. We know little about the first, but it happens during the immune response to an antigen, be it a virus, bacteria, parasite, fungus, or allergen. In this initial response, the immune system produces autoantibodies that stimulate immune cells like mast cells and basophils to secrete inflammatory chemicals. This inflammatory response if prolonged could leave considerable bystander damage in the thyroid gland (Poletaev 2014).

The second wave of antibodies is to clear away damaged antigens or cells that have changed because of the initial encounter. The thyroid autoantibodies that we are discussing are part of the second wave.

This second wave should not be considered a side effect, but rather a reflection of one of the major roles of the immune system—the function of auto-clearance induced by some primary damage of an organ or a tissue (Agapov et al. 2012). Thyrotropin receptor autoantibodies are produced as part of the second wave.

One of the functions of the immune system, although unrecognized, is to regulate the thyroid gland. Now, there is evidence linking the immune system in the regulation of thyroid hormone activity in normal physiological conditions, as well as during times of stress.

Though it's not yet fully understood, they appear to "reflect a process of local intra-thyroidal synthesis of TSH-mediated by a population of immune system cells that traffic to the thyroid." This hitherto undescribed cell population has the potential, to micro-regulate thyroid hormone secretion, leading to critical alterations in the metabolic activity independent of pituitary TSH output.

It has wide-ranging implications for understanding the mechanisms by which the immune system may act to modulate neuroendocrine function during times of host stress (Klein 2006).

We could understand the previous paragraph as expressing the idea that the immune system, during the time of physiological stress, seeks to moderate an overactive thyroid gland by producing TSH-blocking antibodies. However, the purpose of these antibodies is not to destroy the thyroid gland. In fact, "autoantibodies are not damaging to the organism but can have protective functions" (Hampe 2012). They don't cause inflammation either (Grönwall and Silverman 2014; Calabrese et al. 2016). These autoantibodies serve to slow the gland down so that it can heal from the damage caused by the inflammation.

If, on the other hand, the thyroid gland becomes underactive, then the immune system produces thyroid-stimulating antibodies to increase the production of the thyroid hormone. This process happens to the thyroid gland both in normal and stressful conditions.

The consensus in the medical community is that the TSH-blocking antibodies and the thyroid-stimulating autoantibodies are defective. This is nothing more than a non-scientific theory.

Thyrotropin receptor autoantibodies are divided into three groups: activating, blocking, and neutral antibodies, depending on the effect they exert on the thyroid gland. The very names of these antibodies indicate that they are not meant to be destroyers. (the thyrotropin receptor antibodies are regulatory.)

The antibody responsible for hypothyroidism in Hashimoto is called a *TSH-blocking antibody*. The production of these antibodies is not the result of a malfunctioning overactive immune system, but a necessary, normal, restorative, protective, and stabilizing function of the immune system. These antibodies are released when there is an overabundance of thyroid hormone, or the thyroid gland is damaged and needs to be restored.

As the amount of thyroid stimulating hormone blocking antibodies increases in the thyroid gland, the hypothyroid condition becomes worse, but once these autoantibodies are removed, the gland will resume its normal function of producing the thyroid hormone (Hampe 2012).

In Graves' disease, the immune system produces thyroid-stimulating antibodies. These autoantibodies stimulate the thyroid gland to increase the fabrication of thyroid hormones. The production of thyroid-stimulating antibodies is not the result of a malfunctioning immune system, but part of a healthy immune system that is being over stimulated. These autoantibodies are released when there is a short-term need of extra thyroid hormone.

Let me explain: sometimes dust, mold, dander, or pollen gets trapped in the mucous membrane of the throat or nose, causing irritation. The immune system's way of removing the offender is by creating an outburst of air—a sneeze. Sneezing two or three times, to us, is natural. We pay it no attention. But what if the sneezing does not stop? Then we have a problem!

There is nothing wrong with sneezing though! By means of these regulating processes, the immune system helps to maintain the proper level of the thyroid hormone in the body so that all the organs and systems can continue to perform at their peak. The production of these antibodies is meant as a short-term solution to be used in emergency situations. We run into problems when these temporary solutions become chronic.

In most cases, when the immune system directs antibodies at normal cells of the body, they are regulative. They either suppress or stimulate the targeted cell. A prime example of this is the antibodies that attach themselves to basophils and mast cells. They stimulate these immune system cells to produce inflammatory chemicals (Metcalfe et al. 2010). To some degree, it could be argued that the overgrowth of the thyroid gland in Graves' disease is abnormal. However, this abnormality is not because the antibody is defective, but because the production of these antibodies has become abnormal.

Chronic is the keyword. Chronic production of TSH-blocking antibodies will result in hypothyroidism, as in Hashimoto thyroiditis. Conversely, chronic production of thyroid-stimulating antibodies will result in overgrowth of the thyroid gland, as in Graves' disease.

The immune system regulates the thyroid gland via the thyrotropin receptor antibodies, exerting regulating influence on the gland even years after taking treatment for the disease (Klein 2006; Akuzawa et al. 1998). Furthermore, the immune system can produce autoantibodies with the properties of any regulatory molecules in the body and their receptors.

Many experimental and clinical data had directly witnessed that phenomena of this kind are real. Antibodies with biological activity like hormones, autacoids, enzymes and drugs of different classes, have been obtained or registered in patients and healthy donors. According to Klein (2006) and Klein and Wang (2001):

"The immune system is capable of reproducing functional active copies of any biologically active molecule in the body."

For those of us with Hashimoto thyroiditis, this means that the immune system can create autoantibodies with the properties of the thyroid-stimulating hormone, as in the case of Graves' disease. As part of its regulatory ability, it could also produce autoantibodies that block the thyroid-stimulating hormones, as happens in Hashimoto thyroiditis. The immune system creates these autoantibodies due to a biological need.

The question that you may be asking now is this: Why is it that the immune system takes up the mantle as a regulator of the thyroid gland?

The inflammatory chemicals secreted by the immune system interferes with the production of TSH hormones. Considering this obstruction, the backup plan has to be activated, which is: the regulation of the thyroid gland by the immune system. This is the case with Graves' disease.

In Hashimoto thyroiditis, the immune system responds to the disintegration of the thyroid gland due to the inflammation. This process is set in place to help the gland to heal, so, if the inflammation does not stop, neither can this process.

If we really wanted to slow the production of thyrotropin receptor autoantibodies, we could do so by increasing the natural killer (NK) cell population. The NK cells suppress the activity of B cells and, consequently, antibody production. Goji, blueberry, Echinacea, Astragalus, Rhodiola, vitamins (B_{12}, C, and E), beta-carotene, selenium, zinc, curcumin, probiotics, magnesium, and calcium are boosters of NK cells. Green tea and melatonin are known to suppress B cell activity.

At this stage, you do not need to be too concerned over B cells and antibodies. The biggest problem with Hashimoto thyroiditis is not antibodies, but inflammation. Reducing the population of anti-thyroid antibodies is the concern of many. However, once the inflammation has subsided, these autoantibodies will leave the body in secretion, or be broken down by enzymes that degrade protein in the body (Biology Notes with Questions & Answers 2016).

JUICING

There are as many dietary fads as there are differing opinions about them. Some insist that one thing is good and may even swear that it is essential for your health, and then you come across another health professional who contradicts everything the first one suggested.

Often, these people are not very familiar with certain diseases. For this reason, it pays to be well-informed about the different therapies or treatment coming from health care providers. It goes without saying that not all therapies work with all diseases, regardless of how effective they are reported to be. This is especially true when dealing with Hashimoto disease, of which so little is understood.

Juice therapy was one of the treatments that I was recommended, and I found it to be a very concentrated form of delivering nutrients to the body. Some argue against juice drinking because fiber is being excluded, but I didn't consider it necessary to pay attention to that detail. If one's diet is balanced, one can obtain fiber from other sources. At least drinking juice could deliver more nutrients to the body with less energy used.

It is believed that juice therapy is very effective in revitalizing a weakened immune system and creating healthier cells. They also claimed that juice is a very efficient way of delivering nutrients to the body at a cellular level. However, one of the greatest mistakes we make when drinking juice is that we do not permit it to adequately mix with salivary juices, so the first stage of digestion is easily bypassed.

In my experience, juice was not a very helpful therapy for treating Hashimoto disease because it easily lends itself to overconsumption of fructose. Maybe a glass of juice made of orange, beets, pineapple, or any other sweet fruit would not pose any danger if that was all the sugar we consumed during the day. But when we consider the sugar from other sources, much caution is required, considering that we only need about fifty grams or less of sugar daily.

Fructose, the main sugar content in fruits, is healthy and essential for the human body *if* we limited ourselves to no more than fifteen grams of it daily. For those of us suffering from Hashimoto, we cannot overlook the fact that too much fructose over time could have been the cause of the disorder from which we are suffering. If we consume too much fructose, it could damage the lining of the small intestine, causing nutrient absorption problems. This condition is one of the leading causes of gluten intolerance and autoimmune diseases.

Too much fructose consumption also inhibits the cells of the body from absorbing insulin, which then leads to too much of it circulating in the bloodstream. When the brain detects that the cells are not receiving insulin, it releases cortisol to induce the pancreas to produce more insulin, flooding the body with both insulin and cortisol. The excess of these substances in the blood is very damaging to the thyroid gland, so we have a very good reason to limit our ingestion of fructose.

Another reason for cutting down on fructose is that cortisol is also known as the aging hormone. The more cortisol there is in our system, the faster our cells die, and we age.

Juice could also make it very easy for you to over-alkalinize your body, and that can leave you with serious health issues that you don't want to be facing while you're dealing with Hashimoto. If you want to try juices, limit yourself to about four ounces a day.

As a matter of fact, you may experience a turning point in your battle against Hashimoto thyroiditis, just by limiting fructose sugar.

The bottom line for me is that with Hashimoto, drinking juice was not an ideal therapy considering that it could create more problems than it would solve. I found that maintaining a well-balanced diet has always been the best approach.

How is the Thyroid Destroyed?

The thyroid gland is in a war zone; the throat. This zone is one of constant encounters between the immune system and a vast number of antigens, allergens, and pathogens.

Immune system cells are positioned in areas of the body most likely to be visited by enemies. These cells, upon encountering an enemy, release chemicals like histamine with the objective of neutralizing their targeted invader. Even though the intruders may be different, they are all similar in the sense that they induce an inflammatory response from the immune system.

The throat is one of the busiest ports of entry into the body for many of its invaders. We could well describe the throat as the Armageddon of the body. Billions of parasites, viruses, bacteria, antigens, and allergens have met their ends in this killing zone. This is a real burial ground for pathogens. The thyroid, by its location, soon becomes a victim of collateral damage. However, it's not because the immune system directly targets the thyroid gland—it becomes a victim of friendly fire as opposed to fire by mistaken identity.

Abbas and Kumar (1999) states that "For surrounding tissues not to be damaged by inflammatory chemicals, the inflammation must be terminated. This failure will result in chronic inflammation and cellular destruction."

In the inflammatory process, antibodies are like detectives: they identify the intruders and then pass the information on to granulites, which are immune system cells responsible for the initial inflammatory response (Wikipedia 2016). Basophils, mast cells, neutrophils, and eosinophils are cells involved in acute inflammation. These granulites secrete chemicals like histamine, heparin, peroxidase, and chondroitin sulfate in an initial inflammatory immune system response to an antigen. When the inflammation becomes chronic, macrophages and dendritic cells take over and release even more destructive chemicals. So, it should come as no surprise to us if the cells of the thyroid gland, after prolonged exposure to these inflammations-producing chemicals, would at some point succumb and begin to disintegrate.

We could begin the process of recovery by removing the pathogens that trigger the immune system's inflammatory response, whether they are found in our food, or in our environment.

THE STRESS CONNECTION

Hashimoto and stress go hand in hand. They are like Siamese twins. Let's explore this connection to get a better understanding of Hashimoto and be able to escape its deadly grips.

Stress is your body's way of responding to any kind of demand. It can be caused both by good or bad experiences (Mountain State Centers for Independent Living 2016). We all need a little stress in our life to be able to function at an optimal level, but too much stress is unhealthy and should be avoided.

We become stressed when we perceive that something is threatening to pull us out of our comfort zone. According to the Centre for Studies on Human Stress (2016), "Our nervous system cannot tell the difference between a life or death situation, an argument with a friend, a traffic jam, or the monthly bills. It responds to each of these situations in the same way."

There are two types of stress: acute stress, which is a normal part of everyday life, and chronic stress, the repeated exposure to situations that lead to the release of stress hormone.

Chronic stress disrupts almost all the systems in our body. It could shut down the immune system, upset the digestive and reproductive systems, raise blood pressure, increase the risk of heart attack and stroke, speed up the aging process, and leave you vulnerable to many mental and physical problems (Centre for Studies on Human Stress 2016).

Stress could be caused by the good things in life like receiving a promotion, going to college, or buying a house. Sometimes it is brought on by the perception that something may or may not come true, or by irrational pessimistic thoughts (Elkin 2016). Then there are the bad situations such as chronic illness, loss of a job, a death in the family, marital problems, a traumatic event like rape or violence, the list goes on. Our attitudes, perceptions, and expectations, along with our fears and uncertainties, all play a role in stress too (Robinson et al. 2016; WebMD 2016).

Stress is thought dependent. It is the result of the way we perceive something to be. I love the saying by Charles Swindoll, an evangelical Christian pastor, author, educator, and radio preacher, that states: "Life is ten percent what happens to you and ninety percent how you react to it" (1/2CP@cohr 2015).

Something good may happen, but if you perceive it to be bad, that is all it takes to get you started on the downward path of stress. Just one negative thought.

We may be faced with a challenging situation, but it can only stress you if you perceive it to be a stressor.

Allen Elkin (2016) states that "You feel that your stress is the direct consequence of a stressful event or trigger. You may think that 'the situation made me stressed.' And that would be entirely understandable. However, the reality is slow lines, difficult relatives, and loud music don't, in themselves, have the power to automatically make you stressed. You must perceive that situation as stressful. It's your thoughts that are producing your stress."

If we change the way we perceive a situation, our stress levels would be different. The same stresses viewed with a different mindset can result in different feelings. We only need one negative thought to produce that unfavorable stressful environment in our bodies that will open the flow of cortisol and the onslaught of all kinds of unwanted health conditions. The list of potential stressors is long, but, each one of them could only cause stress if we think so.

*If you have Hashimoto
and you are stressed,
your thyroid won't heal.*

In our high-stress culture, the body's stress response center is activated so often that it doesn't have a chance to return to normal, resulting in a state of chronic stress. We must put an end to this madness!

Too much stress will cause fatigue, headache, difficulty falling asleep, frequent waking up at night, mood swings, sugar and caffeine-craving, irritability, light-headedness, dizziness when moving from sitting or lying to a standing position, and gastric ulcers. Stress directly contributes to the body's inability to battle any health condition, especially one as debilitating as Hashimoto (Wikipedia 2016).

There is no pill or medication to lower stress—we must learn to manage it. When the body is submitted to a stressful situation, sickness, viral infection, caffeine, or severe trauma, it releases a complex mix of hormones and chemicals such as adrenaline, cortisol, and norepinephrine to prepare the body for physical action (Chyun et al. 1984).

The initial response is to produce histamine. As stress is prolonged, cortisol becomes the body's weapon of choice. Cortisol is a steroid made by the adrenal glands. Its main function is to increase blood sugar and suppress the immune system, but it also decreases bone formation and helps in the metabolism of fat, protein, and carbohydrates and in the redistribution of glucose (Wikipedia 2016; Glaser and Kiecolt-Glaser 2005; Stress Management Society 2016).

Cortisol takes glucose away from the digestive system and transports it to parts of the body that need it most. The steroid counteracts insulin by making the cells insulin resistant. It also lengthens the time necessary for the healing of wounds and repairing of tissue (Faith et al. 1990).

When cortisol is released into the body, it causes the rapid division of T suppressor cells, while at the same time suppressing the T helper cells. By increasing the number of T-suppressor cells, cortisol prevents the proliferation of T cells, leaving us with a one-sided defensive mechanism relying almost totally on B cells for protection. It's like someone has a stroke and being left with half their body paralyzed (Palacios and Sugawara 1982).

Cortisol functions to reduce inflammation in the body, which is good, but over time these efforts also suppress the pituitary gland's production of thyroid-stimulating hormone and inhibit the conversion of T4 to T3, contributing to hypothyroidism.

Chronic inflammation caused by lifestyle factors such as poor diet and stress helps to keep cortisol levels soaring, putting a strain on the immune system (Castro et al. 2011). An immune system responding to unabated inflammation can lead to a myriad of problems, like increased susceptibility to colds and other illnesses, an increased risk of cancer, the tendency to develop food allergies, an increased risk of an assortment of gastrointestinal issues, and an increased possibility of autoimmune disease (Aronson 2009; Glaser and Kiecolt-Glaser 2005).

During chronic stress, the excess production of cortisol causes fewer receptors to be produced on lymphocytes and macrophages, decreasing tissue sensitivity to the hormone so that inflammation cannot be ended, and altering the effectiveness of cortisol to regulate the immune system response.

When cortisol is not allowed to serve this function, inflammation can get out of control (Virginia Hopkins Test Kits 2016). The abundance of cortisol combined with toxins, allergies, nutrient deficiencies, and other factors provide the ideal atmosphere not only for hypothyroidism but also the development of auto-inflammatory diseases.

Cortisol draws blood from the digestive system and channels it to other areas of the body like the arms, legs, heart, and brain. The digestive system, deprived of adequate amounts of blood, becomes weak and cannot properly digest food. This makes it an easy victim of diseases like celiac disease and food allergies (Carnegie Mellon University 2016; Glaser and Kiecolt-Glaser 2005; Cohen et al. 2012).

For us to have optimal health, it is essential that we have the proper levels of cortisol. Cortisol makes the thyroid gland work more efficiently, but it is not only the thyroid that uses it. Every cell in our bodies has receptors to both cortisol and thyroid hormones (Virginia Hopkins Test Kits 2016; Bennett et al. 2012). High cortisol levels produce resistance to thyroid hormones in the cells and inhibits the production of the thyroid-stimulating hormone. This results in hypothyroid symptoms even if the gland is functioning properly (Trentini 2015).

In our fast-paced, high-stress culture, the adrenals are activated so often, pumping out cortisol, that the body has no time to rest. This causes our body to become over-saturated with cortisol and here is where our problem becomes more critical (Virginia Hopkins Test Kits 2016; Carnegie Mellon University 2016).

Any organ in our body, if exposed to a high level of cortisol over a long period, will succumb to inflammation. In this way, excess cortisol in the blood could start the fire of Hashimoto thyroiditis. If there is too much cortisol in the bloodstream, the thyroid gland will not recover and will remain inflamed.

Although excess cortisol could lay the foundation for Hashimoto, our main problem may not be too much cortisol, but too *little* of it.

As a result of long-term stress, intense exercise, viral infection, caffeine and alcohol consumption, insomnia, and excess sugar, the adrenal glands become exhausted and incapable of producing enough cortisol (Blannin et al. 1999; Biron et al. 2005; Farag et al. 2006; Buxton et al. 1997; Trentini 2015). Where high cortisol levels may lead to a weak immune system, low levels will lead to an overaggressive immune system and the inability of the body to control inflammation.

Hansen (2016) lists the following as negative effects associated with "chronic lower levels of circulating cortisol (as in adrenal fatigue)":

- Brain fog, cloudy-headedness, and mild depression
- Low thyroid function
- Blood sugar imbalances, such as hypoglycemia
- Fatigue—especially morning and mid-afternoon fatigue
- Sleep disruption
- Low blood pressure
- Lowered immune function
- Inflammation

A low cortisol level means that the regulating anti-inflammatory mechanism of the body is absent. Without sufficient cortisol, there is nothing to prevent severe, chronic inflammation. In effect, the immune system is running out of control.

Low cortisol leads to increased production of pro-inflammatory cytokines, proteins that influence the behavior of other cells, which leads to over-activation of the immune system. The result is your body's inability to turn off the inflammatory response. It's like a city without firefighters. The inflammation then starts damaging healthy tissues in your body (Hansen 2016; Reasoner 2013).

Hashimoto thyroiditis is an inflammatory disease. In the absence of sufficient cortisol, there is no way to overcome it. Under such conditions, no treatment protocol for Hashimoto will ever work. This means that bringing your cortisol levels back to normal is not an option, but a requirement.

A low cortisol level is the result of low-functioning adrenal glands. In most cases, this is the result of overuse. You would do yourself a favor if you took your eyes off inflammation or antibodies for a moment and focused it on the adrenal glands.

Any hopes of us recovering from Hashimoto thyroiditis hinges on the return of the adrenal glands to normal functioning. Thus, our nutritional approach should include restoring the adrenals so that the inflammation can end.

Adrenal stress can be caused by anemia, blood sugar swings, gut inflammation, sugar consumption, caffeine intake, excessive alcohol, food intolerance, deficiency in essential fatty acids, environmental toxins, and chronic emotional and psychological stress.

The symptoms of poor adrenal function are lack of energy through the day, fatigue not relieved by sleep, insomnia, difficulty waking up in the morning, feeling lightheaded when standing from a seated position, decreased libido, inability to handle stress, depressed mood, PMS, bad memory, and slow recovery from illnesses (Hashimoto's Healing 2016).

Stress is one of the main factors that can contribute to adrenal fatigue. It is also one of the hardest factors for us to control (Speiser 2016). To keep cortisol levels within the normal range, we need to give our body time to rest and our mind time to relax. We would then be in a better position to see our way out of stressful situations whether they be physical or psychological.

Listen to relaxing music more often, get some massage therapy, laugh a little more. Studies show that just the anticipation of laughter has been enough to reduce cortisol levels. One of the most effective means to deal with stress is by being involved in a contemplative discipline. Get acquainted with your spiritual side (Akedo et al. 2004; Diego et al. 2004; Berk et al. 2008; HowtomakeX 2016).

On the other hand, studies in humans have shown that caffeine increases cortisol and epinephrine at rest and that levels of cortisol after caffeine consumption are like those experienced during an acute stress. Drinking coffee, in other words, re-create stress conditions for the body (Walsh 2016).

A diet containing large amounts of fructose is unhealthier than you probably realized. Fructose not only leads to gradual weight increase, but it also boosts the activity of the stress hormone cortisol. Serbian biochemists have demonstrated this effect in rats that were given fructose water to drink. (Alegret et al. 2007; ergo-log.com. 2016).

Regular sugar is fifty percent glucose and fifty percent fructose, so to reduce fructose intake, you will need to cut down on the amount of regular sugar you consume.

Continuous consumption of alcohol over an extended period has also been shown to raise cortisol levels in the body. *Cortisol* is released during periods of high stress and can result in the temporary shutdown of other physical processes, causing physical damage to the body (Hutchison and Spencer 1999; Wikipedia 2016).

On the nutrition side, the same diet that we use to rebuild the thyroid gland will work just as well for the adrenals. However, it will take about eighteen months to regain full operation of the adrenal glands.

Ashwagandha is proven to heal thyroid and adrenal issues. As an adaptogenic herb, it helps one adapt and deal with stress. It has also been proven effective in supporting adrenal function, helping overcome adrenal fatigue and chronic stress (Dr. Axe 2016). The herb enhances the conversion of T4 to T3, kick-starting thyroid hormone production. It helps treat insomnia, an additional stressor that may cause extra cortisol production, therefore decreasing thyroid function (Demehri 2015).

Cortisol levels that are too low or too high "can lead to regular infections, chronic inflammation, autoimmune diseases, or allergies. Maintaining a balanced level of cortisol is an important part of staying healthy (Hansen 2016).

NOCEBO EFFECT: MIND POWER

The mind is the part of a person that thinks, reasons, feels, and remembers. It is incredibly powerful in that it can heal your body as well as make you sick (Hood 2012).

Our mind is designed to react to impulses of thoughts. Thoughts are just as important to health as the food we eat, the water we drink, or the air we breathe, and the quality of our thoughts is of more importance than the quantity.

Thoughts are electrochemical reactions that stimulate the production of neurotransmitters. They regulate the way the brain functions. This means that thoughts and emotions could exert physical and biological changes in the health of the immune system, for better or worse (MacMillan 2016).

The natural tendency of the mind is to be restless. It is undisciplined and untamed. It constantly jumps from one thought to another in quick succession, allowing thoughts to come and go incessantly, from morning till night, giving us no rest, not even for a moment. These thoughts pop into our minds without permission. They just come, occupy our attention for a moment, and then disappear as others take their place (Sasson 2016).

Many neurological studies have shown that the average person has more than thirty thousand thoughts a day. Of those thoughts, approximately ninety percent are said to be repetitive and eighty percent is classified as negative (Saraswati and Stevenson 2013).

Repetitively thinking about the causes, situational factors, and consequences of one's negative emotional experience can be unpleasant and counterproductive (Marano 2016). When thoughts are reinforced by constant repetition, an attitude is created. Our attitudes influence our bodies, right down to the genetic level. So, the more we improve our mental habits, the more beneficial a response we'll get from our bodies (MacMillan 2016).

Every activity we undertake is part of a creative process. Hashimoto thyroiditis is not a random disease. We manufacture it, one thought at a time.

Most modern-day autoimmune diseases are connected to our brain, so to heal our body, we must first heal our minds (Dalmau and Kayser 2010; Stetka 2015). We have much more power than we imagine; the power to influence our physical and mental realities. Negative thoughts will produce a sick body, and positive thoughts will give us a healthy body. We can tap into the healing and restorative powers that lie within us by changing the nature of our thoughts (Hampton 2016).

If we change our perception of things, we change their outcome. While this is true, the problem for most people is *how* to change negative thinking and the afflictive emotions that are its inevitable consequence (Beliefnet 2016).

Our thoughts have a profound effect on our physical body, spiritual experience, and overall quality of life. The mind, the body and the spirit are all intrinsically interconnected. When one is affected, the other two suffer. We can live a healthy lifestyle and perform our spiritual duties, but the other two cannot make up for the absence caused if the mind is not healthy.

Worry, anger, jealousy, hate, ill will, grudges, vindictiveness, irritation, resentment, guilt, depression, anxiety, lack of joy and happiness and all other negative emotions and thoughts lead to stress, which robs the body of its natural healing capacities. Negative thinking literally wears down the brain and the rest of the body (Gilead Institute of America 2016; McCraty and Rein 2001).

Now there's scientific proof that you can heal yourself and improve your life when you are positive and optimistic. Amazingly, the power of your own thoughts can affect the expression of your genes, and even potentially cure cancer and other diseases (Mercola 2008).

You are what you think: seventy-five to ninety-eight percent of mental and physical illnesses come from our thoughts (Leaf 2011). Every minute of every day, our bodies are physically changing in response to the thoughts that run through our minds. Studies have shown that thoughts alone can change brain chemistry, which could result in less fatigue, adequate immune system reaction, balanced hormone levels, and reduced anxiety (Atasoy 2013).

Just thinking about something causes your brain to release neurotransmitters. There are thousands of receptors in each cell in our body, each receptor is specific to one neurotransmitter. When we have thoughts of anger, sadness, guilt, excitement, happiness, or nervousness, each separate thought releases its own set of neurotransmitters. These surge through the body and connect with their respective receptors, changing the structure of each celle (Debbie Hampton, *how thoughts change your cells and genes*, 2016).

Neurotransmitters are the brain's chemical messengers that communicate information throughout our brain and body. The brain uses neurotransmitters to control all the functions of the body, from hormones to digestion to feeling happy, sad, or stressed.

There are two kinds of neurotransmitters based on functions: inhibitory and excitatory.

Excitatory neurotransmitters are brain stimulants. They are produced by negative thoughts.

Inhibitory neurotransmitters calm the brain, balance the mood, and are easily depleted when the excitatory neurotransmitters are overactive. They are the result of positive thoughts (Boundless 2016).

If the cells are exposed to more excitatory neurotransmitter than inhibitory ones, when they divide, the new cell that is produced will have more of the receptors for the excitatory neurotransmitter than for inhibitory ones. Likewise, the cell will also have fewer receptors for inhibitory neurotransmitters than its mother/sister cell, which was not exposed to them as often (Wikipedia 2016; Thomson 2014).

When you have a perception or a thought of love, the brain releases oxytocin (a hormone that regulates body's metabolism and supports growth), serotonin, and growth hormones. In contrast, when a person is experiencing fear, their brain releases stress hormones (cortisol, norepinephrine, and histamine) that shut down the cell growth process and inhibit the immune system (Biology of Belief 2014).

If you are bombarding your cells with neurotransmitters from a negative attitude, you are literally programming your cells to receive more of these neurotransmitters in the future, making yourself inclined toward negativity. This could prove to be a big problem. (MacMillan, 2016).

It will take more than a few days of positive thinking to make a significant impact on our long-term attitude patterns. If you have a history of negative thinking, depression, pessimism, or perpetual frustration, plan on working on yourself for more than a few days before you see permanent results.

You can start reshaping the biological structure of your cells and become inclined to happiness and optimism instead of whatever emotion you are physically addicted to right now. Adopting positive thinking practices, like mindfulness and gratitude, will change our perceptions of the world and make us feel calmer, more resilient, and happier (Lejuwaan 2016).

Stress is a mental disease with severe physical consequences. If we heal the mind, we heal the body. A sick body is the physical manifestation of a sick mind. In many ways, Hashimoto thyroiditis and many chronic illnesses would not exist if the mind was not stressed.

We used too much energy musing on events in the past, refusing to let go, or perhaps we do not know how. We need to train and discipline the mind to be more productive. This is achieved by instructing it how to think.

The most effective—and maybe the *only* means of training the mind—is the discipline of meditation. This contemplative discipline teaches the mind how to think by training it to let go of unproductive thoughts.

The term *meditation* refers to a process by which we prepare our mind to be more optimistic. Humans are contemplative creatures. Worrying or ruminating is the Western form of Eastern meditation. The sole difference between meditation and worrying is the nature of the thoughts.

Worrying is meditating on negative thoughts.

Many people do everything right. They eat right, exercise, drink water, get enough sunshine, and sleep. Yet they still can't recover from Hashimoto or Graves' disease. Often, this happens because of the *nocebo effect.*

Nocebo is a harmless substance that, when taken by a patient, is associated with harmful effects due to negative expectations or the psychological condition of the patient.

The nocebo effect refers to the fact that your negative beliefs or expectation can result in negative outcomes.

They can make you *sick*. The placebo effect is the opposite, in that positive belief can *heal* you.

Recovering from Hashimoto, as well as from Graves', could be as easy as thinking more positively.

Less thinking is healthier.

You could get much more out of the discipline if you embraced meditation by emptying your mind and thinking more about health, happiness, sharing, helping optimism, beauty, excellence, love, and peace.

We are used to musing on thoughts of death, vengeance, hatred, malice, fraud, hurt, stealing, fear, pain, dishonesty, disappointment, and defeat. Constant contemplation on any one of these is all it takes to put us on the path of stress.

Meditation's purpose is to keep the mind from wandering or worrying. Through meditation, we eliminate the thoughts that cause stress, and with reduction of stress come reduced cortisol levels, improvement in sleep quality, and an overall feeling of well-being.

The procedure is simple. First, find a tranquil place where you will not be interrupted. Forget about the phone or television for that short span of time. You can meditate in any position, anywhere, be it lying down, walking, or sitting.

To begin, fifteen to thirty minutes is an ideal amount of time to dedicate to this discipline. For beginners, sitting down with eyes closed may be the best position to take to prevent distraction.

Meditation tends to place the body in a very relaxed state, so it is advised that the back is well supported. Do not be surprised if you drift into a short nap as that is normal.

Now choose a word or short phrase about something pleasant—a positive thought. Slowly repeat that phrase and immerse yourself in the beauty and pleasantness of it. Don't permit any other thought to intrude on this moment. Just savor it. Keep concentrating on your chosen word or sentiment for the entire duration.

In the beginning, this may feel like a waste of time, but after a few days, you will begin to see and feel the difference, so do not quit. Join a community of people who indulge in the art of meditation. You may also want to spend more time in the woods, gaze at the stars, listen to the waves, spend time in the garden, stop and smell the roses or lilies, or just listen to the birds. Whatever it takes, pursue a contemplative lifestyle, because, in the solitude of contemplation, you will find healing.

Many helpful attitudes—such as forgiveness, gratitude, and kindness—can be cultivated through the discipline of meditation and mindfulness. (Krull 2016).

Mindfulness is a state of active, open attention on the present. When you're mindful, you observe your thoughts and feelings from a distance, without judging them as good or bad. Mindfulness means living in the moment and enjoying the experience (Psychology Today 2016).

Mindfulness and regular meditation practice have been proven to be immensely valuable in shifting negative thought patterns and brain activity.

THE ALLERGY FACTOR

Allergy is one factor that cannot be ignored when dealing with Hashimoto thyroiditis.

Allergy is caused by a hypersensitivity of the immune system to something in the environment that usually causes little or no problem in most people. Some diseases that result from allergies are hay fever, food allergies, atopic dermatitis, allergic asthma, and anaphylaxis (Wikipedia 2016; WebMD 2016). Symptoms may include red eyes, an itchy rash, a runny nose, shortness of breath, or swelling.

We all experience reactions to allergens, but not to the same degree. Our tolerance is determined by our lifestyle, genes, and the environment. Some of us have a very high tolerance to certain chemicals while others may have a low threshold. This is the reason why some people manifest allergic reaction to certain food or toxins while others don't.

An allergic reaction is dependent on two things: tolerance to an allergen, and tolerance to histamine in the bloodstream.

Our bodies have tolerance levels of all chemicals to which we are exposed whether they are found in food or in the environment. The fact that everyone does not exhibit identical symptoms of a substance is no indication that they do not have an immune system response to the same chemical. The reaction may just have been lower in intensity.

If someone consumes a considerable amount of certain food consistently over a long period, there comes a moment when certain proteins in that food will breach the barrier of tolerance and provoke an allergic reaction.

A low tolerance level means we experience a maximum reaction while a high tolerance level means a minimum reaction. For us to experience an allergic reaction, the immune system must do two things: create basophils and mast cells, and produce antibodies, a type of protein called immunoglobulin (Metcalfe et al. 2010).

The basophils and mast cells are distributed over the entire body but are mostly concentrated in areas that interact with the outside world. These include the nose, lungs, skin, gastrointestinal tracts, and throat (therefore allergic symptoms will be more pronounced in these locations than anywhere else in the body).

When an allergy-inducing agent is encountered, it triggers the B cells of the immune system to produce antibodies in large quantities. These antibodies attach themselves to the basophils and mast cells. When these cells encounter an allergen, they degranulate, releasing histamine and other allergy-causing chemicals in abundance (City Allergy 2016).

Substances that can cause allergic reactions are called *allergens*. Examples of these are pollens, dust mites, molds, animal proteins, foods, and medications. When an allergic individual encounter an allergen, histamine is the chemical secreted in a larger amount. It produces different symptoms depending on the part of the body where it is released. Everyone may react to allergens; however, allergic symptoms may not be visible because the histamine created is not enough to produce symptoms.

In some cases, allergic reactions may be caused by foods that have not been properly broken down by digestion, cooking, or enzymes. When this happens, it is usually referred to as *food intolerance* and the effects are mostly felt in the digestive system.

Some proteins, if consumed even in a small amount, will induce adverse reactions in our bodies, provoking an immune response. An example of this is Ara h2, the most important allergen in peanuts (Ertmann et al. 2004). Other foods contain chemicals that, in small amounts, are harmless, but in larger quantities become toxic to us. These will also provoke immune system reactions. (A prime example of this is with gluten.)

When the immune system interacts with allergens consistently over a long period, it contributes to the inevitable chronic inflammation, which could lead to diseases such as Hashimoto thyroiditis.

There are two stages of an allergic response: the immediate phase which could last up to ninety minutes, and the late phase that can last up to twenty-four hours. If the immediate phase and the late phase merge, then we could have a severe allergic reaction.

When an allergen is detected, the mast cells secrete their mediating chemical histamine, and an inflammation is produced in the general area. After the initial response, other immune cells—eosinophils, neutrophils, and lymphocytes—are recruited to the site. Once they've arrived, each one of these cells contributes to the late phase of the allergic response. Eosinophils generate chemicals like those made by mast cells, but they also release more generally toxic substances that irritate the body. Neutrophils release many chemicals, including enzymes, which degrade protein, and in turn, causes further tissue damage (City Allergy 2016).

If this allergic encounter happens in the throat area, often the inflammation will cause deterioration and eventual destruction of the cells of the thyroid gland. Thyroid hormones and other components will then leak into the bloodstream. The longer the exposure of the thyroid to these chemicals, the more extensive the damage, and, consequently, the more hormones and proteins that escape into the bloodstream, activating the immune system into action by producing thyroid autoantibodies.

Clinical tests may say that you have no allergies, but, most people have an immune system reaction to these allergens. These reactions may be so mild that they are not worth further attention in normal individuals. When you do an allergy test, the doctor may casually mention the antigens to which you have a mild allergic reaction and affirm that there is no need to be concerned about them. However, we should make it our responsibility to identify all allergens to which we react and if there is inflammation of the thyroid, do our best to avoid them.

In Hashimoto thyroiditis, these mild reactions could be key contributing factors in prolonging the illness. But, because these allergens are not on our suspect list, we ignore them and find ourselves unable to heal.

About human-friendly chemicals: just because an immune system reaction to that chemical is mild, it does *not* mean it is human-friendly. For example, we have gluten. Data obtained from a pilot study support the hypothesis that gluten elicits its harmful effects on all individuals (Arranz et al. 2006; Thompson 2001), which means that everyone is allergic to gluten to some degree.

There is an enzyme in the blood called *transglutaminase*. When combined with gliadin, it enhances the immune-stimulatory effect of gluten (Corazzaa et al. 2012). The body can neutralize gluten in small quantity, but that is no indication that gliadin is harmless (Fleckenstein et al. 2004).

All humans have these reactions, but not all of us are affected equally. Why? Because we experience allergic reactions only when the histamine levels in our body become too much for our system to handle.

Excessive consumption of certain types of foods, such as wheat, over a long time will cause the levels of gliadin to increases in the body. At some point, this excess of gliadin will induce our immune system into producing histamine.

The immune system is very effective in doing its job, but if we continue to feed on these histamines-producing substances day in and day out, the histamine levels will continue to increase until the organs and systems of the body consequently begin to fail. Consuming too much histamine-producing food could be enough to lay the foundation for Hashimoto.

Once we've contracted the disease, even the mildest allergic reactions to any allergen could prevent improvement. These reactions might have gone undetected or unnoticed (if there was only one), but when combined in a group with other mild allergic responses, a chronic condition could develop or deteriorate.

All allergens—regardless of the source—produce histamine, and all allergic reactions are caused by excess histamine, so any substances that induce histamine production, however mild, could propel the body over the tolerance limit of the said substance, triggering an allergic symptom.

Histamine

Solving the problem of inflammation of the thyroid gland is fifty percent of the solution to Hashimoto thyroiditis. The other fifty is rebuilding the gland (Milas 2014).

Inflammation of the thyroid gland could be caused by chemicals, viruses, bacteria, or fungus. Inflammation is how the body responds to infections. It is supposed to be short-lived, not to last for an extended period (Nordqvist 2015). When the body fails to eliminate the cause of inflammation, it could persist for weeks, months, and even years, resulting in chronic inflammation.

I invite you to look at one of the leading causes of inflammation: histamine.

Histamine is a chemical compound naturally occurring in food and drink. It is found in all human tissues and certain cells of the immune system, mainly in basophils and mast cells. It forms part of the body's protective mechanism against foreign invaders and is used as a neurotransmitter or messenger in the brain.

During stress or physical injury, the immune system releases histamine and other inflammatory substances. They rush to the damaged area and cause the blood vessels to widen to facilitate access of the white blood cells to the area of injury where they could fight off bacteria and start the healing process (Mandal 2014).

When we become exposed to airborne toxins such as pollen, animal dander, dust mites, molds, spores, and ragweed, histamine is released into the respiratory system. This causes swelling, to reduce the volume of air inhaled and limit exposure to these airborne toxins. It also produces coughing, a protective reflex to clear the trachea and bronchi, helping to expel mucous fluids, and with them, allergens that have settled in the upper and lower airways. The release of too much histamine in the lungs could lead to asthma (White 1990).

As we can see, histamine is very beneficial to the human body. With the help of the enzyme diamine oxidase, it's easy for us to quickly assimilate dietary histamine. When the levels of diamine oxidase go too low, histamine rises above the tolerance level, leading to histamine intolerance (Maintz and Novak 2007). Vigilance then becomes a requirement, especially if Hashimoto thyroiditis is involved.

The foods naturally rich in histamine are tomatoes, spinach, eggplants, avocados, mushrooms, strawberries, bananas, papaya, kiwi, pineapples, mango, prunes, peas, sunflower seeds, peanuts, and tree nuts (Histamine Intolerance 2016).

Food from animal sources contain very little histamine; however, they are rich in the amino acid histidine. As these foods are stored, bacteria convert histidine into histamine. The longer the meat is aged, salted, smoked, dried, or marinated, the greater the content of histamine produced. In contrast, fresh food contains less histamine (Diet-and-Health.net 2016).

The following fermented foods are very high in histamine content: vinegar, soy sauce, cheese, mustard, ketchup, alcohol, red wine, white wine, champagne, beer, pickled and canned vegetables, sausages, ham, salami, pepperoni, and bacon (Paleo Leap 2016). We should also be aware of citrus fruits, like oranges, grapefruits, tangerine, and limes; they also have a high histamine content.

Some food contains tyramine, which, once consumed, induces mast cells and basophils to produce histamine without the intervention of the immune system. Tyramine-containing foods are fish, especially tuna, mackerel, sardine, catfish, salmon, and herring. Foods also on this list are chocolate, coffee, black tea, bread, and other products with yeast (Ede 2016).

Drugs such as penicillin, sulfa, and aspirin cause the release of histamine. Too much estrogen also stimulates the production of this compound. Mastocytosis, an overabundance of mast cells and bacterial infection, can contribute to the increase of histamine levels.

The biggest non-food source of histamines in most people's bodies is their gut flora. Some bacteria produce histamine while others degrade them. Good gut flora is important if you want to keep your histamine levels down (Paleo Leap 2016).

All immune system reactions to allergens result in the production of histamine. Unfortunately, histamine is virtually indestructible outside of the body. It cannot be destroyed by cooking, baking, canning, smoking, boiling, freezing, or roasting. Once it has been ingested, our bodies can easily break it down if it has enough diamine oxidase. When this enzyme is depleted, we develop food sensitivities and allergy symptoms (Ede 2016).

Regardless of the source of histamine—whether it be from stress, allergenic proteins, bacteria, food, medications, or too many mast cells—the result is always the same: digestive problems, stomach cramps, diarrhea, acid reflux, headaches, skin rashes, eye itch, nose itch, skin itches, rashes, watery eyes, congested sinuses, wheezing, excess mucus production, hives, spasms, and anxiety. When we take into consideration, that histamine is so readily available, even if your allergy test result is negative, you could still experience allergy symptoms if the histamine levels in your body go beyond the threshold of tolerance.

Too much histamine is one of the leading factors in chronic inflammation of our organs and tissues, including that of the thyroid gland. Excess histamine, also leads to suppression of the immune system, because it reduces the activity and production of T cells, sending us deeper into a B cell–dominated immune system. (Nancy Khardori, Rahat Ali Khan, Trivendra Tripathi - 2010)

If you are someone who often experiences allergic reactions or regularly find yourself in the need to purchase antihistamines to mask allergy symptoms, and you have Hashimoto thyroiditis, you may just have discovered one of the sources of your inflamed thyroid gland.

An antihistamine may grant a temporary relief from the effects of allergies or excess histamine, but do not be fooled! Antihistamine medication will *not* contribute to improvements in any autoimmune disease because, like most medications, they only put a mask on the symptoms but do not stop the production of histamine or reduce its levels.

Here is a partial list of the side effects that you could experience from taking antihistamines: dry mouth, drowsiness, dizziness, nausea, vomiting, restlessness, moodiness, trouble urinating or not being able to urinate, blurred vision, confusion, and constipation.

It makes me wonder, what is the point of taking antihistamines if you are going to be suffering all these side effects?

Obviously, we can't stop eating all histamine containing and producing food because then we would literally starve. All we need to do is manage the amount of histamine we consume.

All foods have the potential to increase the level of histamine. As histamine levels increase, so does the potential for inflammation. The higher the level of histamine goes above the level of tolerance, the greater the damage will be to the organs and tissues of the body.

The sad reality of modern-day living is that histamine in our body is hardly ever below the tolerance level, so we experience an allergic reaction to foods that do not even contain allergens.

If you are someone who listens to their body, and you are afflicted with an autoimmune disease, this could easily be verified. You may eat a certain food one day and experience an allergic reaction, and the following day you eat the same food, but everything is normal. Why is that so? It's because allergic reactions don't depend on specific allergens, but on histamine levels. It is abundant in the food we eat, so we could easily go over the limit even if we have no significant issue with allergens.

Have you ever wondered why a peanut allergy is so devastating? Peanut has eleven allergenic proteins, and each one of these allergens will have an immune system response, causing the histamine levels in the blood to skyrocket. This could have serious health-threatening consequences. Peanut is dangerous because its histamine-producing potential is so great.

Everyone has a different tolerance level, and there is no median tolerance level established for histamine, but one thing is sure: for most people with Hashimoto thyroiditis, if they could maintain the histamine in their body below their own tolerance level, it would improve their chances of recovery. This should be one of the first steps to consider as you embark on your journey to recovery.

The main causes of allergic reactions are eating too much histamine-containing and histamine-producing foods, allergen-containing foods, intoxicating polluted foods, and genetically engineered foods.

Histamine by itself has the potential to be the root cause of Hashimoto thyroiditis because it could both cause the thyroid gland to become inflamed, and at the same time, suppress the immune system. Anyone who suffers from Hashimoto should not ignore the role that histamine plays in causing this condition to deteriorate, even if the inflammation is caused by something else like medication, infections, cortisol, or gluten.

There are tests to measure the histamine level in one's blood. However, our histamine level changes daily depending on the food we eat. Unless you do a test every day, it would not be very helpful. A more effective approach is to become familiarized with the effects of histamine in your body and use these symptoms as your guide.

An anti-Hashimoto diet is exactly what we need in our struggle to contain Hashimoto thyroiditis. Avoid histamine-producing food as much as possible and eat foods that contain elements that fight inflammation. Some of these special foods are apple cider vinegar, lime or lemon juice, ginger, quinoa, Ashwagandha, bee pollen, hemp seed, and cinnamon. All these contain powerful anti-inflammatory agents and are also immune system boosters, regulators and anti-allergic.

You could never go wrong by doing a self-test, which is the same procedure that one undergoes in an effort to determine allergic reactions to foods. First, you would want to restrict (or better yet, abstain from) foods that have a high content of histamine. This process is more effective when done at night, because when the body is at rest, it is easier to feel the effect of food on the body as it is assimilated into the system. It works by eating the suspect food for supper. If it causes no reactions, put it on the list of foods that are safe to eat.

For this experiment, only one item of food should be consumed at a time. Of course, you could also eat more than one kind of food, if you are one hundred percent sure that you are not allergic to the other food items on the menu. I would recommend testing each item of food for two or even three nights, especially if you feel any adverse reaction. Obtaining the same result two or three times should be enough evidence for it to be crossed off the list of foods to eat.

Anytime that the inflammation flares up in the thyroid gland, it may produce the following symptoms: increase of energy during the night (enough to cause insomnia), accumulation of mucous in the throat area, an increase in body temperature (sometimes enough to cause sweating), and mild hoarseness. These symptoms may last for one to three hours depending on how much food was consumed. The symptoms in the morning would be a sense of weakness, drowsiness, and a somewhat sore throat.

If you do this test early in the onset of the disease or during the later stages of remission, these symptoms would be almost unrecognizable. Do not make that mistake of ignoring them because of their mildness—every bit counts.

Also, with the thyroid gland functioning normally, some of these reactions would be of no consequence. But with an already underactive thyroid gland, anything that worsens its function could be easily detected and should be avoided like a plague. After the inflammation has subsided, these foods could be slowly and moderately re-introduced back into the diet with no negative consequences.

I did an allergy test, which turned out negative. However, I noticed that I had a mild sensitivity to nuts and sometimes grains, so I decided to put myself in a process of food elimination. The interesting detail about these mild reactions is that they contribute to the disease. In eliminating these mildly reacting elements from your diet, you will experience a noticeable improvement in your condition.

Putting everything into perspective, excess histamine by itself could cause Hashimoto thyroiditis. For some people, just properly managing the level of histamine is enough to send Hashimoto thyroiditis into remission. Then again, allergies or histamine may not be the main cause of the inflammation but may be one of the leading contributing factors.

THE POWER OF SLEEP

Often, we sacrifice the time that we should dedicate to sleep, to accomplish more in life. Sometimes, we look at sleeping as just a pastime. However, rest is one of the natural laws of health (Amazing Discoveries 2016). We cannot overlook rest when dealing with Hashimoto, especially given the fact that being able to sleep becomes a big problem for victims of Hashimoto thyroiditis.

If the body cannot obtain enough rest, it will never recover from any illness. We permit ourselves to fall prey to the idea that by getting less sleep, we could accomplish more, but we could never be further away from the truth. Our bodies need time to recover from illnesses, restore energy, repair damaged organs and tissues, and fight off invaders. We must then make a conscious effort to provide our bodies with this needed time of rest to give ourselves the best chances of recovery.

The habit of having a big meal immediately before going to bed impacts our quality of sleep. When we have supper, especially close to bedtime, almost all the organs of our body must work overtime. Some of these organs should be resting and not working. This habit leaves us feeling tired the next morning even if we appear to have slept.

One of the main reasons for sleeplessness is the consumption of foods that contains allergens (National Sleep Foundation 2016). As the allergen is absorbed into the bloodstream, it produces inflammation in different parts of the body, and the thyroid gland is one of the most common victims. The inflammation caused contributes even more to the already compromised gland. Its cells disintegrate, leaking thyroid hormone into the bloodstream. This hormone is used to produce energy, and although this energy may not be a lot, it is often enough to cause sleep to disappear. Even very small amounts of an allergen could have this effect.

The very chemicals produced by allergens cause sleeplessness, even in the absence of inflammation of the thyroid gland. If the thyroid gland was normal, the effects of some allergens would go unnoticed, but with an inflamed, underactive gland, the slightest undesired reaction from the food we ingest is easily felt. So, to enjoy a better night's rest, avoiding all allergens at supper time is suggested.

Another reason for sleeplessness is too much cortisol in the body, released by the adrenal glands during stressful situations. Cortisol has the unique property of making it impossible for the body to rest.

Consuming too much fructose could have the same effect on our sleeping habits as fructose induces the production of cortisol.

Caffeine-containing drinks like coffee and colas may contribute to the production of cortisol. Bryan Walsh, of Precision Nutrition (2016), says that "Studies in humans have shown that caffeine increases cortisol and epinephrine at rest and that levels of cortisol after caffeine consumption are like those experienced during acute stress. Drinking coffee, in other words, re-creates stress conditions for our bodies."

Sometimes our sleeplessness is due to a deficiency in sleep-inducing nutrients, such as L-tryptophan. This amino acid is found in turkey, fish, oats, beans, lentils, eggs, dairy products, and some fruits, the best source of which is the banana. So, eating protein-rich foods could prove to be helpful. The recommended daily intake of tryptophan is four milligrams per kilogram of body weight (HealthAliciousNess 2016).

A very good sleep snatcher is watching TV right up to bedtime. It is a perfect recipe for poor quality of sleep as sometimes we cannot get those vivid images out of our minds to be able to rest. Watching TV promotes the production of cortisol as well, and the brain needs at least one hour for the cortisol level to diminish to the point where the sleep mechanism could kick in (National Sleep Foundation 2016). Watching TV also hinders the secretion of melatonin, a hormone necessary for sleep quality (Schultz 2013).

The bottom line here would be to turn off the TV a couple of hours before bedtime and to engage in a brain-relaxing exercise such as reading or meditation.

Remember that quantity of sleep is also important. Most of us, under normal circumstances, need about eight hours of sleep every day, yet those of us who have Hashimoto or regular hypothyroidism undoubtedly need more time because our body does replenish itself at a slower pace than when normal.

Sleeplessness is an immune system suppressant, so one can argue that suppressing the immune system in the case of Hashimoto is supposed to be a good thing because our problem is an overactive immune system. That is *not* the case! Suppressing the immune system by depriving ourselves of sleep is counterproductive. As victims of this autoimmune condition, we need at least nine hours of sleep a night, so let's not cheat ourselves and strive to get more sleep.

Sleeplessness could also be caused by an over-acidic or over-alkaline body, which makes it more imperative that we learn to balance out our diet.

The quality of our sleep could also be compromised if we drink too much water close to bedtime. Waking up too many times during the night to go to the washroom could cost you in terms of health, so give yourself time to rest!

As you can see, there are many factors that may contribute to sleepless nights. This means that obtaining a good night's sleep becomes very challenging at best.

THE DIGESTIVE SYSTEM

There is an emerging consensus among health care providers that ultimately, digestive health shapes the immune system. It is therefore important to understand how the digestive system is connected to immunity.

Data shows that the digestive tracks are host to 70 percent of the immune tissue in the body and that a compromised intestinal barrier plays a role in the development of autoimmune diseases like Hashimoto. So, it is in our best interest to obtain a good understanding of the factors involved in having a healthy and strong digestive system (koyuncu A).

It is the digestive system's responsibility to separate all the raw material that we eat and prepare them for metabolizing. This process involves removing toxins, separating nutrients, and killing off invading bacteria, parasites, and viruses. The digestive system makes sure that everything is prepared and ready for use. The system does its job adequately if it is provided with the proper raw material, which comes in the form of food.

Digestion starts as soon as the food hits the mouth where saliva begins the process of breaking it down. Once it reaches the small intestine, vitamins, minerals, carbohydrates, enzymes, and other substances are absorbed into the bloodstream through microscopic pores in the intestine's lining and transported into the cells of the body. These pores limit what enters the bloodstream, working like a sieve that filters out undesirable substances.

Sometimes, these pores become irritated and inflamed, causing the pores to expand and break. This allows toxins, undigested food, and larger molecules to enter the bloodstream.

Two possible causes of this irritation are an imbalance between good and bad bacteria, and the presence of too much lectin, or toxin, in one's diet. Other causes could be medication, radiation, chemotherapy, long-term use of aspirin, and antibiotics.

However, of interest to Hashimoto victims is the issue of low stomach acid, identified as a co-factor in the onset of autoimmune diseases.

According to Jonathan Wright, MD, author of "Why Stomach Acid is Good for You," approximately 90 percent of Americans produce too little stomach acid. He arrived at this conclusion after measuring the stomach pH of thousands of patients in his clinic (Katy Haldiman, MS, RN).

Low stomach acid leads to imbalanced gut flora, bloating, gas, belching and constipation. The predominant belief is that these symptoms are caused by having too much acid in the stomach. However, doctors are beginning to realize that low stomach acid is the common overlooked cause (Steve Wright).

When functioning properly, the parietal cells of the stomach secrete hydrochloric acid bringing the stomach acidity to a range between 1.5 and 3.0. The stomach is separated from the esophagus by the Lower Esophageal Sphincter (LES). When the stomach acid reaches to the proper level, which normally takes about 20-30 minutes after eating, it signals the LES to close tightly, so that food digestion can take place without harming the esophageal lining. However, when stomach acid levels are low, it does not give off the closing signal, and the LES remain open.

There is also the pyloric sphincter that separates the stomach from the small intestine which allows the food to exit the stomach into the small intestine. But, the body will not open the pyloric sphincter if the contents of the stomach are not properly acidified. So instead of moving through the pyloric sphincter into the small intestine, food sits in the stomach and ferments, producing gas and pressure. As the intra-abdominal pressure of digestion increases, it pushes against the LES which gives way because it was never really closed in the first place. Acidic stomach fluid or fumes comes back up into the lower part of the esophagus causing a burning sensation; commonly referred to as heart burn.

The inner lining of the stomach is protected from its own acid by a thick layer of mucous and epithelial cells that produce a bicarbonate solution to neutralize the acid. But, even a microscopic amount of stomach acid touching the inside of the esophagus will produce pain and burning. This is because the esophagus is not protected like the stomach from high acidic chemicals (Katy Haldiman, MS. RN).

When the stomach is not able to produce enough acid to bring down the pH level of the food to an optimal range, the trigger to release sodium bicarbonate which neutralizes the stomach's acid is not activated. The high pH of the food also fails to trigger the release of pancreatic digestive enzymes and bile necessary to further breakdown the carbohydrates, proteins, and fats. This leads to food sensitivities, allergies, inflammation, and autoimmune disease (Katy Haldiman, MS. RN).

Poor diet, stress, the consumption of processed foods, refine sugar and age contributes to decrease stomach acid production, setting the stage for illness and disease. You could eat plenty of protein and still be protein-malnourished if you have low stomach acid (Bajaj et al., 1979), (Krasinski et al., 1986).

There are several disorders associated with insufficient stomach acid, among those are: Addison disease, asthma, celiac disease, diabetes, eczema, chronic autoimmune disorders, food allergies, gall bladder disease, gastric cancer, gastritis, graves' disease, hepatitis, lupus, osteoporosis, pernicious anemia, psoriasis, acne, rosacea, thyrotoxicosis, urticaria, vitiligo, colitis, hair loss, multiple sclerosis and rheumatoid arthritis. (Nutrition review).

Low stomach acid can lead to over-growth of pathogenic bacteria, like the *Helicobacter pylori* or *H. pylori*, which has been found to be common in people with Graves disease and Hashimoto and can lead to gastritis (Rafsanjani et. Al., 2003), (STTM 2003).

A research study has established that "People with Hashimoto have decreased production of gastric acid, because of the slowing down of the metabolism (Ebert EC)."

The interconnectedness between the hormonal and the digestive systems is amazing. It makes sense why Nobel Prize-winning Physician Dr. Mechnikov is quoted as saying, "Death begins in the colon." (Duke J. A).

You can't have a healthy gut without a healthy thyroid, and you can't have a healthy thyroid without a healthy gut. To restore proper function of the gut-thyroid axis, both must be addressed simultaneously.

Thyroid hormone conversion is dependent on healthy digestion. Inflammation in the gut reduces T3 by raising cortisol. Cortisol decreases active T3 levels (Stockigt, JR and Baverman LE). You could see why this is a dilemma for Hashimoto sufferers.

The answer to low stomach acid is not using over-the-counter antacids which can neutralize stomach acid and make your digestion worse. The key to improving your digestion is in increasing your stomach acid by:

Eating plenty of mineral-rich vegetables (Rafsanjani et al., 2003)
Reducing consumption of sugar, especially fructose.

Chewing: it sounds too simple, but digestion starts in the mouth. Chew foods thoroughly to stimulate digestive enzymes in the mouth and break up foods into the smallest particles possible for better digestion.

Peppermint is used to aid the various processes of digestion due to its antibacterial and gastric-acid-promoting properties. Peppermint also aids digestive function by combating gas, increasing the flow of bile, and healing the stomach and liver (Schilcher, H, Deutshe Apotheker Zeitung).

Vitamins: The nutrients needed for healthy thyroid function are B12, vitamin A, vitamin E, B vitamins, selenium, iodine, zinc, iron, and magnesium. As the digestive problem gets worse, so does the thyroid problem because these nutrients are not present in optimal levels. Eating foods rich in these nutrients will help improve thyroid function.

Zinc is essential to produce stomach acid. Most foods that are high in zinc are animal foods such as beef, lamb, crabmeat, turkey, chicken, lobster, clams and salmon. Zinc food sources aside from meats are dairy products such as yogurt, kefir, cheese, nutritional yeast, peanuts, beans, wholegrain cereals, brown rice, whole wheat bread, and potatoes. Pumpkin seeds are the most concentrated, non-meat food source of zinc. Vitamin C, E, B6, and minerals such as magnesium help increase zinc absorption in the body.

Proper combination of food makes digestion easier. Protein requires stomach acid to be digested and carbohydrates reduce the production of stomach acid, so do not eat proteins and carbohydrates/starches together. Instead, pair proteins with low-starch vegetables. Protein and fats go well together because they stimulate the liver and gall to produce bile and dump it into the small intestines. Good fats like coconut oil, palm oil, olive oil, fish oil, and flaxseed oil. Starches/carbohydrates with vegetables are a good combination, but fruit should be eaten alone—not with meals because they lower the production of stomach acid.

Ice water with meals is not recommendable because it inhibits production of stomach acid and slows down digestion. If you would like a drink with your meal, try adding warm ginger tea, which increases the production of stomach acid (Branch Basics).

Squeeze ½ of a lemon in a glass of water and sip on it while eating. Lemon juice can help supplement the acid in your stomach, aiding digestion. Additionally, this mixture can help decrease bloating and abdominal gas (Garnett Cheney 1949).

Bitters stimulate stomach acid secretion, pancreatic enzymes and increase bile from the gallbladder. When possible, eat dandelion greens or other bitter herbs with meals.

Two of the best natural solutions to low stomach acid are cabbage juice and Apple cider vinegar.

Cabbage is an excellent source of vitamin K, vitamin C, and vitamin B6. It is also a very good source of manganese, dietary fiber, potassium, vitamin B1, folate, and copper. Additionally, cabbage is a good source of choline, phosphorus, vitamin B2, magnesium, calcium, selenium, iron, pantothenic acid, protein and niacin (George Mateljan).

You probably have not heard about vitamin U. That is because it's not actually a vitamin at all. It is a name used to describe a healing enzyme found in cabbage. (Collective Evolution).

When stomach acid has been chronically low for years, the stomach lining may be inflamed and unable to tolerate acid supplementation. In this case, vitamin U is useful in soothing the inflamed stomach lining and correcting low stomach acid (Garnett Cheney 1949).

The most common way to consume it is in liquid or spray form, but it can also be taken in tablet form or directly from foods. The richest natural sources of vitamin U are cabbage, alfalfa sprouts, spinach, kale, tomatoes, celery, wheat, turnips, radishes, and parsley.

Drink four ounces of cabbage juice with meal. It works well in both children and adults that are free of any hypothyroid problem. If you have Hashimoto, do not use the cabbage. Your best option is using the extract, vitamin U. (Garnett Cheney 1949)

Raw Apple Cider Vinegar: There are a few theories regarding just why apple cider vinegar improves digestion and low stomach acid. First, the vinegar is acidic and will lower the acidity in the stomach. Frequent doses of raw apple cider vinegar are also reported to be effective in correcting Candida overgrowth, and Candida problems can contribute to low stomach acid production. It is very effective as a quick solution when one is experiencing heartburn, a sign of low stomach acid.

Upon waking, drink 1/2-1 tsp. raw apple cider vinegar (it must be raw) in 1/2 cup warm water. Take this solution before each meal and if needed after meals to stop heartburn (Lauren 2013).

THE LIVER

The human adult liver weighs about 3.1 pounds, is in the right upper abdomen, below the diaphragm. Liver tissue is made up of smaller units called lobules. Blood coming from the digestive organs flows through the portal vein to the liver, carrying nutrients, medication and toxic substances. The liver converts the toxic substances it receives into harmless ones and safely escorts them from our bodies (liver.ca).

The benefits of a healthy liver are increased energy, clear skin, regular menstrual cycle, freedom from sinus pain, fewer infections, strong immunity, less digestive complaints, fresh breath, positive mood and a sharp mind.

The liver helps to ensure that the level of blood glucose stays constant. It also produces bile, stores and regulates vitamins, minerals, and amino acids from foods, so that they can be used to produce energy, or make glucose and fat (Pubmed health 2016).

It processes everything you eat, drink, breath, or rub on your skin. Every day, the liver helps the body with fighting infections, eliminating toxins, clothing the blood, regulating hormones, neutralizing poisonous substances, balancing insulin, sex hormones, thyroid hormone, cortisone, betatrophin and in producing and regulating cholesterol.

According to health researchers at University Park, Pa., an excess of bacteria in the gut can change the way the liver processes fat and could lead to the development of metabolic syndrome (Victoria M. Indivero 2015).

A metabolic syndrome is a group of conditions including obesity, type 2 diabetes, high blood pressure, high blood sugar and excess body fat around the waist. Research published in the February 2007 issue of the *Journal of Clinical Endocrinology and Metabolism* established a connection between thyroid function and metabolic syndrome (Roos, Annemieke, et al.)

What the researchers found was that in those with normal TSH levels and slightly low thyroid hormone levels, but still within the normal range, had significant increased the risk for developing metabolic syndrome (Huang et al., 1995).

This is interesting because the liver plays an important role in thyroid hormone metabolism. 60 percent of thyroid hormones (T4) are converted into the usable (T3) form in the liver. Hypothyroidism interferes with liver function causing fewer thyroid hormones to become active, leading to symptoms of fatigue, brain fog, joint pain, hair loss, weight gain, and depression.

If you can learn how to heal your liver, then your thyroid function will improve drastically.

The liver processes a lot of sugar in the form of glycogen. Thyroid hormone controls this hepatic glycogen synthesis, so when one is afflicted with Hashimoto Thyroiditis, the liver's ability to produce glycogen is reduced, paving the way for the development of blood sugar issues (Bollen M, Stalmans W).

When you can't balance your blood sugar, the body begins to produce glucocorticoids; these stress hormones then begin to break down healthy muscle tissue and converting them into sugar to keep your brain functioning. However, these hormones also block the liver from converting thyroid hormone into its active T3 form. (Heyma P and larkins RG)

Another problem that can develop is estrogen dominance and the autoimmune form of hypothyroidism called Hashimoto's thyroiditis, if this female hormone is not broken down efficiently. Estrogen affects thyroid by directly blocking the thyroid gland from releasing thyroid hormone. Estrogen also promotes the production of thyroid suppressive stress hormone and inhibits or slows down metabolism (Wang et al.).

Memory, mood, and blood sugar are linked to estrogen build-up. The role of estrogen in hypothyroidism is well-researched. To get the thyroid back in working order, it is necessary to address estrogen.

The bile produced by the liver with the help of dietary fiber, work together in eliminating excess estrogen and other waste from the body. When the liver is not working at an optimal level, you run the risk of having estrogen build up to toxic levels, or the body may store them in fat.

This is where **carrot** comes to the rescue. Raw carrot is made up of a unique fiber that absorbs excess estrogen and helps escort it out of the body. Carrot fibre binds to estrogen and keeps it from being absorbed in the intestine, then helps to safely escort it out of the body. Raw carrot fibre also helps to lower the number of endotoxin-producing bacteria. These bacteria create an additional burden for the liver, keeping it from doing its regular job of processing and eliminating excess hormones (Ray Peat, PhD).

The Gall Bladder

The **gall bladder** is a pear-shaped sack, located on the right side of the abdomen under the liver. Its primary function is to store and concentrate bile; a yellow-brown digestive enzyme produced by the liver. The bile contributes to the digestive process by breaking up fats. It also drains waste products from the liver into the small intestine.

Proper bile flow and production also help us with proper judgment, clear thinking and decision making. When we have Liver/Gall Bladder issues, we may not think things through before acting, or we may become indecisive.

A sluggish gall bladder interferes with proper liver detoxification and prevents hormones from being cleared from the body. Many people with Hashimoto thyroiditis have gall bladder issues because low thyroid function slows down the flow of bile from the gall bladder, which can lead to slower breakdown of fats, cholesterol and toxins in the liver. This sluggish and congested process also contributes to the formation of gall stones.

The number one cause of liver damage in the industrialized world is lifestyle habits. They include: eating refined process food, too much sugar, alcohol, and caffeine, prescription medication or antibiotic use, low-quality animal products, high-stress levels, environmental toxins and the use of chemical household and beauty products.

A nourishing diet is the best way to keep your liver healthy and functioning the way you need it. We must learn to educate our taste buds to enjoy eating real, whole foods, vegetables, fruits and healthy fats. This diet will influence how well the liver works.

Ginger: contains chemicals that have been shown to increase bile secretion and reduce cholesterol levels.

Garlic, just a small amount of this pungent white bulb could activate liver enzymes that help your body flush out toxins. Garlic holds high amounts of allicin and selenium, two natural compounds that aid in liver cleansing. Garlic has long been regarded as powerful antimicrobial agents that lower inflammation in the liver while increasing circulation and healthy blood flow. Take note that garlic in high dose has the potential ability to induce liver damage but low doses (0.1 or 0.25 g / kg body weight/day) are safe (Rana SV et al., 2006).

Fruits like berries and melons provide the balance electrolyte minerals needed by the liver, like magnesium, calcium, and potassium. Grapefruit is high in antioxidants; it increases the natural cleansing processes of the liver. Apples are high in pectin and other chemical constituents necessary for the body to cleanse and release toxins from the digestive tract (Dr. Edward Group DC, NP, DACBN, DCBCN, DABFM 2015).

Bitter foods: Bitter green vegetables, mustard greens, bitter gourd, chicory, arugula, dandelion, collards and Swiss chard, raise levels of glutathione and are loaded with nutrients and probiotics. Bitter foods also stimulate the liver to produce bile, which is an important part of optimal digestion. Bile emulsifies fats and makes nutrients, especially fat-soluble ones such as vitamins A, D, E, and K, more available (Dr. Andrew Weil 2014).

Lemons & Limes, these citrus fruits contain very high amounts of vitamin C, which aids the body in converting toxic materials into substances that can be dissolved in water.

Turmeric is the liver's favorite spice. Turmeric contains curcumin, a compound helpful in restoring healthy blood pressure, improving circulation and fighting toxin buildup (Lai HS, et al., 2005).

We need a detoxified liver to avoid inflammatory autoimmune reactions, food allergies, and sensitivities or leaky gut syndrome. When it comes to liver health and detoxification the best approach is, choosing high-antioxidant foods to flush toxins out. Curcumin fits those qualifications (Klein AV and Kiat H. 2015)

Herbs including turmeric, coriander, parsley, cilantro, and oregano are great to improve liver health and boost glutathione production and lower inflammation.

Raw honey, the kind that's not heated or refined. It is a natural antibacterial, antimicrobial and antifungal product. It helps lower liver inflammation and eliminates bacteria, parasites, and viral infections. Honey contains a diverse array of nutrients, including B vitamins, calcium, potassium, magnesium and vitamin C.

Raw honey also contains amino acids, which are the building blocks of protein. Perhaps most interestingly, honey contains phenolic compounds, which are beneficial substances that possess antioxidant properties. It also nourishes the digestive tract, improves gut health and protects the liver from toxic substances (Janet Renee Ms. RD 2015).

Apple cider vinegar: The benefits of apple cider vinegar come from its powerful healing compounds which include acetic acid, malic acid, potassium, magnesium, probiotics, and enzymes.

Acetic acid kills unwanted bacteria as soon as it encounters them, making it a natural antibiotic, while at the same time it fosters the growth of beneficial bacteria.

Apple cider vinegar naturally provides numerous benefits related to skin, digestion, and immune health without any side effects. It balances the pH level within the body, which enables the liver and other organs to work optimally (Dr. Axe).

Milk thistle is the richest *source* of *silymarin*. In fact, *silymarin* is often called milk thistle extract because its seeds contain about 70 percent of the phytonutrient, according to the Encyclopedia of *Natural* Medicine. But it can also be found in artichoke, coriander, and turmeric. There are also trace amounts in grapes, beet greens, peanuts, brewer's yeast and berries (Carlos Mano).

This herb increases the solubility of bile and has been shown to significantly lower cholesterol concentrations in the gall bladder. It has potent anti-oxidant activity which supports detoxification and it prevents depletion of glutathione in the liver, which is often depleted in people with Hashimoto's. It also has anti-inflammatory properties, and it promotes protein synthesis in replacing damaged liver cells.

Milk thistle strengthens the liver cells wall, buffering them from invading toxins, supports liver regeneration and glutathione formation. In this way, salymarin works to benefit diabetics.

Milk thistle is considered safe and well-tolerated, with very few cases of side effects ever reported. The most common side effects aren't serious and include a mild laxative effect.

When taken within the recommended dose range, milk thistle is thought to be effective and mostly free of allergic reactions and interactions (Post-White J et al. 2007).

Consumption of the oral form of milk thistle at 420 mg/day in divided doses is considered safe for up to 41 months, based on clinical trial data (Drugs.com milk thistle).

Panax ginseng: This herb has been shown in several studies to have numerous positive impacts on liver function. It has been shown to reverse fatty liver in animals and can be helpful in cleaning toxins out of the liver. It also has important benefits for the immune system like promoting Kupffer cells (specialized immune cells located in the liver).

Relaxation: The liver in traditional Chinese physiology oversees the smooth flow of life energy throughout the body, any disruption in its functions usually affects other organs. Stagnation of the flow of liver *energy* frequently disrupts the emotional flow, producing feelings of frustration or anger. These same emotions can lead to dysfunction in the liver, resulting in an endless loop of cause and effect (Bill Schoenbart and Ellen Shefi).

Research shows that stress promotes inflammatory responses and worsens liver damage, even contributing to liver diseases. It's no longer a speculation that stress impacts the liver and hormones; it's now been proven. A contemplative discipline would be a health promoting addition to your life (Chida Y, Sudo N. and Kubo C. 2006).

Exercise helps blood and nutrients reach reproductive or digestive organs, helping to bring on a healthy, more pain-free menstrual cycle and regular bowel movements. Exercise training benefits the management of obesity-related liver diseases even if you do not experience any weight reduction. Particularly, these effects seem to be acquired through an improvement in the liver inflammatory condition and its related oxidative stress levels. The liver is then better able to release blood to the brain, organs, tendons, joints and muscles (Oh S. et al., 2013).

Selenium is necessary to support and activate the conversion of thyroid hormone in your liver. Selenium deficiency is a common trait among Hashimoto sufferers. It is not something that should be ignored, so make sure you're getting an adequate amount in your diet. Some of the best sources include: shrimp, cod, scallops, and mushrooms (Arthur et al.).

Foods to avoid in favor of good liver health include: too much alcohol or caffeine, refined vegetable oils, artificial ingredients, sweeteners and food coloring, non-organic crops, factory-farmed animal products, farm-raised fish or conventional dairy, sugary drinks and snacks and refined grains. Crops sprayed with chemicals, farm-raised fish or factory-farm-produced meat/poultry; they are more likely to carry toxins, antibiotic residue and added synthetic hormones that are sure to overtax the liver to remove them.

THE ENDOTHELIUM

The endothelium is made up of 6 trillion cells that line 100,000 miles of blood vessels in a single layer throughout the body.

Endothelial cells are the weak link in the circulatory system. They form a thin layer, only one cell thick, which lines the insides of the arteries. They are regulators of nutrient uptake from the blood and are instrumental in blood pressure regulation (Byron J. Richards).

Endothelial cells are the major producer of Nitric Oxide, the critical molecule responsible for relaxing the blood vessels and maintaining healthy blood flow. Since healthy nitric oxide levels are crucial in maintaining a healthy heart, focusing on the endothelium, is an important part of supporting long-term wellness (Dr. Louis Ignarro).

The vascular endothelium is the primary site of dysfunction in many diseases, particularly cardiovascular disease. A variety of risk factors, including smoking, hypercholesterolemia, hypertension, and diabetes Mellitus, adversely affect endothelial function.

When the liver is damaged by pollution, excess alcohol, medications, street drugs, and excess food, the endothelial cells lining the circulatory system within the liver, orchestrate the rejuvenation process.

Endothelial cells within liver enable stem cells to form new liver cells and then coordinate the linking together of the liver cells to form new organ structure. As the amounts of stress, chemicals, toxins, pollutants, antigens, and other irritants meet them, they run the potential risk of damage.

When endothelial cells are damaged, new endothelial cells are produced in the bone marrow and travel to the liver or anywhere else to fix the injured area. This implies that bone health must be maintained to have a good supply of rejuvenating endothelial cells.

Researchers have demonstrated that this mechanism of liver organ rejuvenation likely applies to all organs and glands, including the thyroid. So, the concept of preserving the health of your endothelial cells to aid general organ rejuvenation is a fundamental principle of health (Laurie D. DeLeve 2013).

Evidence has emerged suggesting that the best way to keep the endothelial cells healthy is to limit saturated fats and eat a balanced diet that includes fresh fruits and vegetables, whole grains, lean protein and low-fat dairy. Omega-3 fatty acids, antioxidant vitamins, especially vitamins C and E (tocotrienol), folic acid, and L-arginine, L-citrulline, silymarin, taurine, and grape seed extract, appear to have beneficial effects on vascular endothelial function (Allison A Brown and, Frank B Hu 2001. Dr. Louis Ignarro).

Nitric oxide is a molecule that our body produces to help its 50 trillion cells communicate with each other by transmitting signals throughout the entire body. Nitric oxide has been shown to be important in helping memory and behavior by transmitting information between nerve cells in the brain and to assist the immune system at fighting off bacteria and defending against tumors. Nitric oxide regulates blood pressure by dilating arteries, reducing inflammation, improving sleep quality, and Increase your recognition of sense (i.e. smell), increasing endurance and strength to assist in gastric motility (*Jason Clark, BSc, MSc*).

The most common way to increase nitric oxide is through exercise. When you run or lift weights, your muscles need more oxygen which is supplied by the blood. As the heart pumps with more pressure to supply the muscles with blood, the endothelial cells in your arteries releases nitric oxide into the blood, which relaxes and widens the vessel wall, allowing for more blood to pass, though. As we age, our blood vessels and nitric oxide system become less efficient due to free radical damage, inactivity, and poor diet, causing our veins and arteries to deteriorate.

Nitric oxide is produced through diet, most notably by consuming the amino acids L-arginine and L-citrulline. Arginine, which can be found in nuts, fruits, meats and dairy, directly creates nitric oxide and citrulline inside the cell. Citrulline is then recycled back into arginine in the kidneys, making, even more, nitric oxide. These enzymes that convert arginine to citrulline and citrulline to arginine need to function optimally for efficient nitric oxide production. We can protect those enzymes and nitric oxide by consuming healthy foods and antioxidants like fruit, garlic, soy, vitamins C and E, Co-Q10, and alpha lipoic acid, allowing the body to produce more nitric oxide. Nitric oxide only lasts a few seconds in the body, so the body must be constantly producing it. This means that the more nutrients and antioxidants we can provide the body; the more stable nitrite oxide will be and the longer it will last.

Since arginine levels become depleted during exercise, the entire arginine-nitric oxide - citrulline loop can lose efficiency, causing less-than-ideal nitric oxide levels and higher lactate levels. Supplements can help restore this loop allowing for better workouts and faster recovery from workouts

Many of the studies published so far suggest that subclinical hypothyroidism accelerates endothelial dysfunction. Hypothyroidism is associated with increased of LDL-cholesterol, diastolic blood pressure, and markers of chronic inflammation and simultaneously reduces the bioavailability of nitric oxide to blood vessels.

Another study published in the Journal of American Heart Association reveals that Hypothyroidism in women is associated with microvascular endothelial dysfunction. This may explain some of the increased risk of cardiovascular disease in people with Hashimoto (Jaskanwal et al.)

Exercise

Exercise provides the body with extra energy and can result in a longer life. We were never designed to remain sedentary. The human body was created for action and it functions better when in constant motion (Chamberlin 2009).

The comforts of our modern society have converted us into a highly sedentary species. Deprived of movement, our organs become paralyzed and unable to function. Inactivity is described by the Department of Health as a silent killer. The evidence is emerging that sedentary behavior like sitting or lying down for long periods is horrible for your health (National Health Service 2015).

We reason that we could function without exercise, unaware that in doing so, we become active contributors to illness. Lack of physical activity contributes to approximately seventeen percent of heart disease and diabetes cases, twelve percent of falls in the elderly, and ten percent of breast and colon cancer cases (Silberner 2010).

Exercise increases the number of endorphins, a natural hormone, in the body that produces a sense of well-being and increases the quality of sleep. Both Hashimoto and stress are promoters of sleeplessness, just one more reason for us to include exercise in our daily routine. Exercise is also an immune system booster, helping to induce and increase the productivity of the thyroid gland.

Exercise also relaxes blood vessels, lowers blood pressure, reduces muscle tension, and helps in relieving both physical and mental stress (Breene 2013; WebMD 2016). It has also been shown to partially reverse the effects of the aging process on the physiological functions.

It can reduce the risk of premature death and inflammation in the body (Kistler et al. 2012).

However, while exercise is beneficial, too much of it could be detrimental. When one has Hashimoto, everything in the body marches virtually in slow motion, as all the organs and systems of the body perform at a lower rate than normal. The thyroid does not manufacture enough hormones, so heart rate and blood pressure are lower than usual, the brain's performance capacity is diminished, and the liver, kidney and the rest of the body's organs work in a manner that is below average. Because of this if we stress the body by doing more than it can handle in its current weakened condition; muscles will begin to secrete chemicals which must then be cleared out of the body by the kidneys. Taking into consideration that the kidneys are already compromised, they can become overloaded, malfunction, and begin to die.

You want to be moderate in your exercise program. Thirty minutes a day of moderate walking, three to four times a week, is all that is needed.

All in all, it is almost impossible to recover from Hashimoto thyroiditis without regular exercise. So, try *really try*, to fit it into your regiment.

LECTIN AND YOUR HEALTH

Lectins are a class of carbohydrate-binding proteins found in all forms of life, including human. Lectins are used to achieve many basic functions in the body, like cell-to-cell adherence, managing inflammation, program cell growth, death and fat modulation.

Lectins are a part of plants natural defense mechanisms, vital for seed survival. Some plant lectins are beneficial to humans; however, two classes of lectins are known to be problematic to the human body.

The first are called prolamins because they are rich in the amino acid, proline; gluten is the most prominent example of a prolamin. The second group tends to clump red blood cells together, so they have been called agglutinins. Prolamin and agglutinin lectins are found to some degree in all foods and they have considerable potential to cause serious health issues if not monitored closely.

Lectins are sticky molecules that binds to human tissue, especially intestinal cells, kidney and adrenals in susceptible individuals, allowing the possibility for developing subclinical conditions, which appear over time and are usually considered being of unknown origin (Krispin Sullivan, CN 10/05/16).

Lectins are also called *anti-nutrients* because they are toxic substances. They can affect the turnover and loss of gut epithelial cells, damage the Luminal membranes of the epithelium, stimulate shifts in the bacterial flora and modulate the immune state of the digestive tract. Lectins can also promote enlargement or the wasting away of key internal organs and tissues and alter hormonal and immunological balance (Vasconcelos IM and Oliveira JT. 2004).

As lectins circulate in the body, they can bind to any tissue like the thyroid, pancreas or collagen in joints. This binding, disrupt the function of that tissue and cause immune system cells to attack the lectin-bound tissue, destroying both the lectin and the tissue. This autoimmune response, lead to disease (Pusztai A. 1993).

The stickiness of lectins allows them to bind to the gastrointestinal lining, particularly the villi, of the small intestine, disrupting the everyday wear-and-tear that occurs in the intestine, gradually leading to a reduced absorption of nutrients. The constant consumption of lectins, prevent these villi from regenerating as fast as they need to keep the intestinal lining secure, leading to intestinal permeability commonly known as leaky gut (Greer Fand Pusztai A. Katsuya Miyake et al., 2007).

Studies show that Lectins are involved in food allergies, food sensitivities, and inflammation, by inducing the discharge of histamine from gastric mast cells. It's no coincidence that the top 8 allergens also contain some of the highest amounts of lectins. These are dairy, egg, wheat, soy, peanuts, tree nuts, fish and shellfish (Ryan Andrews; Science Daily)

Of interest to many, is the implication of lectins in the progression of hypothyroidism. Lectins stimulate class II HLA antigens on cells that do not normally display them, such as pancreatic islet and thyroid cells. Class II HLA is a genetic coding signal that informs the immune system that the cell has been infected. The lectins that can have this effect are found in tomato, wheat, potato, peanut, and soy. There is a strong possibility that Hashimoto is a lectin-driven disease (David L J Freed and Allergist 1999), (Uchigata Y et al., 1987).

Other foods contain proteins similar in chemical composition to gliadin and could be just as destructive to the body if we consume them in very large quantities. Barley has hordein, rye has secalin, corn has zein, oat has avenin, and milk has casein. The allergen in seafood has been identified as parvalbumins, and in plant food, including nuts, grass, and weed, the allergen is profilin. Be temperate when consuming them.

Wheat Gluten

Gluten gives the wheat grain its elasticity and chewing property, it is also one of the main triggers of the inflammation that damages the thyroid gland.

As time progresses, more and more people are becoming gluten intolerant. This may be due to the intense genetic modification to which wheat grains have been subjected over the years. Today's wheat plants have been genetically manipulated to produce more yields, and it contains significantly more gluten than they did thirty years ago.

Furthermore, the gluten found in modern wheat owes much of its DNA to one of the goat grass with which traditional wheat was crossed. This gluten was desirable because of its elasticity and pliability. On a cellular level, our bodies simply don't recognize this modified protein. This paired up with the fact that it also contains an appetite stimulant, poses a big problem for us; it causes us to eat more (Treehugger 2016) (Modern Wheat is bad for you 2016).

Our digestive system was designed to handle a little gluten, but the exaggerated amount of gluten contained in food today, damages our intestinal tract, making it impossible for proper digestion and absorption of nutrients. The immune system, in an effort protect the body from this invader, produces inflammatory chemicals with the intention of neutralizing it, subsequently eliminating the threat with no side effects when the amount of gluten consumed is within a certain limit.

Our body can neutralize all the chemicals contained in the food we eat if they are consumed in moderate amounts. A good deal of health-threatening substances are easily disposed of without us being aware of their presence in our bodies, but when the intake of these chemicals is above what the body can handle, they become toxic to our organs and systems. It is then that we begin to see and feel their effects in the form of allergic symptoms. Sometimes these chemicals cross-react with other substances in the body and produce toxic by-products as well, which may provoke immune system reactions.

Gliadin and aglutenin are the two main components of gluten. Bloating, gas, abdominal pain, headache, fatigue, anemia, osteoporosis, infertility, joint pain, vomiting, and difficulty breathing are just a few of the health problems related to the consumption of gluten. Hashimoto thyroiditis is one more addition to the long list of evils attributed to consuming wheat thanks to gluten and, more specifically, gliadin.

The data obtained from many studies; support the hypothesis that gliadin is not harmless by any stretch of the imagination. Gliadin is a toxic substance that, in and of itself, will execute considerable damage to muscles, systems, organs, and tissues of the body, beginning with the intestines (D Bernardo et al., 2007).

Gliadin damages the cerebellum which could cause disorders such as the inability to coordinate and balance body movements and problems with speech, as in the case of autism. It stimulates appetite, inducing people to eat more so they could become obese.

Other brain disorders that have been associated with gliadin are schizophrenia and epilepsy. It could also cause bone loss, impaired hearing, and dermatitis. Gliadin damages the pancreas, liver, and gall bladder, all of which help the body to produce digestive chemicals and enzymes. When these organs are compromised, the digestive process begins to break down, becoming ineffective.

Gliadin is threatening to the health of the human body.

Gliadin has no health-promoting properties. As soon as it enters the body, our immune system reacts to it. This battle between gliadin and the immune system, if prolonged, will lead to celiac disease, Hashimoto thyroiditis, and many other ailments.

Wheat Germ Agglutinin

Wheat germ agglutinin lectin can damage any tissues in the human body without a genetic susceptibility. Even in the absence of intolerance or allergy to wheat or gluten. Wheat germ agglutinin may just be the invisible enemy in many chronic inflammatory and degenerative conditions; the silent killer among the wheat-consuming populations.

According to Nutrition educator Sayer Ji, "wheat germ agglutinin lectin is exceptionally hard to get rid of as it is formed by the same disulfide bonds that make vulcanized rubber and human hair so strong, flexible and durable. Wheat germ agglutinin lectins are extremely small, resistant to breakdown by living systems or organisms and tend to accumulate and become incorporated into tissues where they interfere with normal biological processes," (Educator – Sayer Ji).

Wheat germ agglutinin is very small; it can pass through the cell membranes of the intestine with ease, even in the absence of celiac disease or leaky gut syndrome. Having gained access to general circulation, these lectins may bind to surface cell membranes in arteries and vessels, organs and glands, including the thyroid and pancreas. You do not need to eat a lot of wheat germ agglutinin before they become a problem. The inflammatory process in our bodies could be stimulated into being by an exceedingly small concentration of wheat germ agglutinin (Chiara Dalla Pellegrina et al.).

Studies have demonstrated that wheat germ agglutinin is toxic to both normal and cancerous cell and capable of inducing either cell cycle arrest (stop replication) or programmed cell death (Liu WK et al., 2004).

Wheat germ agglutinin has also been shown to have an insulin-like effect on the cells of the body, so the victims continue to increase in weight and insulin resistance. Wheat germ agglutinin also inhibits the production of secretin, interfering with digestion which can cause pancreatic hypertrophy (Yevdokimova NY and Yefimov AS. 2001).

Secretin is a digestive hormone released into the bloodstream by the duodenum in response to acidity, to stimulate the pancreas to secrete pancreatic juice. The wheat germ agglutinin lectin has been shown to inhibit secretin production by about 57 percent (Mikkat U. et al., 1998).

Wheat germ agglutinin is extremely bioactive on immune cells as it has been shown to induce histamine secretion from mast cells and is also capable of directly stimulating monocytes and macrophages. It can both initiate and maintain inflammation in the body (Food democracy 2013).

Wheat germ agglutinin can alter the integrity of the epithelium layer as they are designed to bind to specific carbohydrates that project off the surface of cells.

The two glycoproteins with which wheat germ agglutinin have the greatest affinity, are *N-AcetylGlucosamine* and *N-Acetylneuraminic acid.*

N-acetylglucosamine is a very specific form of amino sugar (glucosamine) that binds the disruptive wheat lectin. This form of amino sugar is very effective at lectin-binding. One of N-acetylglucosamine most interesting abilities is its function to suppress the anti-secretin effects of the wheat lectin (Mikkat U. et al.,1998).

N-Acetylglucosamine is also involved in the structural integrity and production of cartilage, tendons, and joints.

Glycocalyx is a mucous secreted in humans by the epithelial cells which line all the mucous membranes from nasal cavities at the top to the gastrointestinal tract at the bottom as well as the protective and slippery lining of our blood vessels. The glycocalyx helps the body differentiate between its own cells, disease cells, and invading organism. The glycocalyx is made up largely of N-Acetylglucosamine and N-Acetylneuraminic acid (Sietze et al., 2007).

If we consume too much wheat germ agglutinin, we could exhaust our supply of N-Acetylglucosamine and N-

Acetylneuraminic acid and find ourselves deprived of the protection offered by glycocalyx.

N-Acetylneuraminic Acid and *N-Acetylglucosamine* is found in abundance in whey protein isolate. Eggs are also a very good source of N-Acetylneuraminic Acid and N-Acetylglucosamine. For those who are unable to incorporate enough of these dietary sources, these substances can be found in supplement form as well.

Potato lectin

Solanine is a plant toxin found in species of the nightshade family, such as potato, tomato, and eggplant. It can occur naturally in any part of the plant, including the leaves, fruit, and tubers. Solanine is indeed a poison in large doses, causing everything from gastrointestinal symptoms to hallucinations, paralysis, and death (The BMJ 1979 Dec 8).

According to Harriet Hall from 'science based medicine', one would have to eat about 20 kilograms (44 pounds) of potatoes at one meal to die from solanine intoxication. So, there is no need to be concerned about potato lectin (Harriet Hall).

Have you ever wondered, how many kilos of potatoes have you eaten in the last ten or twenty years? Solanine is a slow killer; it is only a matter of time before it gets you. So, you better get to it first.

You may think that the amounts of lectin specifically solanine in potatoes are probably way too low for it to be of any real concern, however, think again! The problem for many people is that their body cannot break down solanine. The solanine then builds up in the major organs, including the liver, thyroid gland and skeletal muscles and can cause all sorts of problems.

Solanine is an alkaloid merged with a sugar. When the body begins to metabolize solanine, the sugar separates and solanine gets absorbed into the circulation. While not immediately toxic in the amounts ingested from nightshade vegetables, solanine can be stored in the body, so it accumulates and becomes a slow killer; a source of stress and detriment in the body (W. D. B. Claringbold et al.).

The glycoalkaloids in potatoes including solanine are known to contribute to Irritable Bowel Syndrome and negatively affect intestinal permeability (Sayer Ji, Founder).

Solanine and the other nightshade steroidal alkaloids can irritate the gastrointestinal system and act as acetylcholinesterase inhibitors, preventing it from breaking down acetylcholine, thereby increasing both the level and duration of action of the neurotransmitter acetylcholine (McGehee DS, et al., 2000).

Acetylcholine is a chemical messenger that triggers muscle contractions and stimulates the excretion of certain hormones. In the central nervous system, it is involved in wakefulness, attentiveness, anger, aggression, sexuality and thirst, among other things (The brain from top to bottom).

Once acetylcholine does its job, it must be rapidly broken down into acetate and choline by another chemical substance called cholinesterase. When there is not enough cholinesterase, it results in accumulation of acetylcholine which causes continuous stimulation of the muscles, glands, and central nervous system. This can result in fatal convulsions (Dell DD and Kehoe C.1996).

If you have Hashimoto, the recommendation is: to reduce your consumption of potatoes, at least until the disease is under control.

Dairy Lectin

Cow's milk is thought to be an environmental trigger for the autoimmune response in Type 1 diabetes. There is ample evidence that some children who are fed cow's milk at a young age may become allergic to casein, a protein found in cow's milk (Harrison LC and Honeyman MC. 1999).

The story goes that some 5,000 years ago, a mutation occurred with the *proline* amino acid, converting it to *histidine*. Proline has a strong bond to a small protein called β -*casomorphins* 7 (BCM 7), which helps keep it from getting absorbed into the body. Histidine, the mutated protein, binds on to BCM 7, but it has a weak hold. So, as they go through the gastrointestinal track, BCM 7 is liberated and absorbed into the blood of animals and humans who drink A1 cow milk.

Cows that have this mutated beta casein are called A1 cows and include breeds like Holstein (Russian Breakthrough Unravels BCM7 Mysteries).

BCM 7 has been shown to cause neurological impairment in animals and people exposed to it. Dr. Woodford's book "Devil in the Milk" presents research showing a direct correlation between a population's exposure to A1 cow's milk and incidence of autoimmune disease, heart disease, type 1 diabetes, autism, schizophrenia, organ damage, and malfunction of the gastrointestinal tract. Too much of these substances may affect the thyroid gland. If you are aware of a current thyroid problem, it is best to avoid food that contains A1 casein (Russian Breakthrough Unravels BCM7 Mysteries)

Genetically modified organism

Genetically modified organisms are plants, animals or microorganisms, in which the genetic material has been altered in a way that does not occur naturally. Genetic modification is achieved mostly by splicing lectins.

Foods are often genetically modified to make them more resistant to disease, improve nutritional value, or increase their ability to grow in different climate conditions.

Researchers have been experimenting with inserting the gene from lectins normally found in one species of plant or micro-organism into other species as a way of increasing their resistance to pests or disease.

Lectins are chosen for their natural toxic characteristics. This is how pest resistance is transferred; by splicing a lectin from a pest-resistant species into one that is not. When lectins are transferred to a food plant that is normally healthy, this adds additional lectins to the number of naturally occurring lectins in the food plant, contributing to the bad effects lectins exert on the human population (David Peterson, DC, DCCN, FAAIM).

In North America, it's impossible to eliminate lectins from the diet altogether and you cannot avoid genetically modified foods. According to a report by Dr. Oz, more than 80 percent of the foods we eat on a daily basis contain one or more types of genetically modified organism. What you can do is scale down dramatically on the foods that are the most problematic for Hypothyroidism, eat a variety of foods and place a lot of effort on intestinal health (*JP. et al.* 2009).

Lectin Solution

Although all foods contain some lectins, only about 30% of the foods we eat contain them in significant amounts. Legumes (including beans, soybeans, and peanuts) and grains contain the most lectins, followed by dairy, seafood, and plants in the nightshade family. It is estimated that about five percent of the lectins we eat will enter circulation (*Am J Clin Nutr* 1980 33: 11 2338-45).

Five percent does not sound like a lot, but don't be fooled; humans are very vulnerable to the toxicity of lectins. Concentrated amounts can cause digestive issues and long-term health problems. In fact, lectins are highly resistant to the body's digestive enzymes and can easily pass through the stomach unchanged (Heshmati J and Namazi N. 2015).

The most extensively studied lectins are called phytohemagglutinins, which are mostly found in plants, especially legumes. Raw legumes, like kidney beans, are the biggest sources of these lectins. Eating raw kidney beans can lead to lectin poisoning, the main symptoms of which include severe abdominal pain, vomiting, and diarrhea (Noah ND et al., 1980).

Cooking, soaking or sprouting seeds and grains helps to degrade lectins and other anti-nutrients in foods. Fermenting the foods can also work, by allowing friendly bacteria to digest the anti-nutrients (Yang F et al., 2001; Singh AK et al., 2015).

However, not all lectins are destroyed by these methods, and some particularly stubborn lectins remain no matter how lengthy the treatment. *In some cases, the lectin activity is enhanced by sprouting (like alfalfa sprouts).*

Thus, these techniques don't totally reduce the negative effects for everyone.

Wheat germ contains one of the types of lectin that isn't destroyed during digestion, so the body often produces antibodies to get rid of them. Our responses to dietary lectin vary, but almost everyone has antibodies to some dietary lectins in their body (Tommy Jönsson et al.).

Blood Type

Some health care providers insist that knowing your blood type is an important tool for understanding how your body reacts to food, your susceptibility to disease, your natural reaction to stress, and so much more (Stephany Watson 2016).

Based on this theory, a blood type diet has been proposed. Proponents of this diet suggest that your blood type determines which foods are best for your health. Let us take a closer look at this diet.

People who are type A should eat a plant rich diet completely free of red meat; in other words, a vegetarian diet. Foods that they should avoid are Lima beans, Tomato, Eggplant, and Garbanzo bean.

Lectins from certain foods could be harmful to some blood types, but at the same time, be beneficial for others. In the case of blood type, A, the lectin in soy can help the immune system keep guard against cellular changes that could go on to be problematic (Glycobiology)

Type B people can eat plants and meats except for chicken and pork, and can also eat some dairy. However, they should avoid wheat, soy, corn, buckwheat, lentils, tomatoes and a few other foods.

Type AB could partake of seafood, tofu, dairy, beans, and grains. But kidney beans, fava beans, corn, beef, bell pepper and chicken could be problematic for them. Also avoid caffeine, alcohol, and smoked or cured meats.

Type O is a high-protein diet based largely on meat, fish, poultry, some fruits, and vegetables, but limited in grains, legumes, and dairy. Wheat, Soy, Peanut and Kidney bean could be very harmful to these people. Wheat germ agglutinin, the most common lectin found in wheat, binds to the lining of the small intestine, causing substantial reactions and irritation in some blood types – especially Type O (Gerhard Uhlenbruck, Ph.D., MD).

Simply put, when you eat a food containing lectin protein that is not compatible with your blood type, the lectins pass through the gut wall and enter the circulatory system where they target the organ and system of your body and begin to agglutinate blood cells in that area. Some lectins, particularly those found in common grains, are especially attracted to the body's fat cells where they bind to the insulin receptors on these cells. Once bound to the receptors, they signal fat cells to stop burning fat and store extra calories as fat. So, they promote insulin resistance (D. Adamo).

Various research shows that most agglutinating lectins are not necessarily blood-type specific, except for a few varieties of raw legumes; they react with **all** blood types. However, some lectins will have a more profound effect on a specific blood type than on the others (Lajolo FM and Genovese MI 2002).

In contrast, there is also strong evidence that people with certain blood types can have a higher or lower risk of contracting certain diseases. Maybe it has something to do with the lectins in foods. Different diets work for different people. Although there is no conclusive evidence to support the blood-type diet as it relates to Hashimoto Thyroiditis. Keep an open mind, there may be something to it (Yamamoto F, et al. 2012).

If your current diet is not working, it may be time to try a blood type diet; it may just work for you.

Mucin

Mucin: Some people have problems with lectins, but just don't know it. Often, the problem with lectins is only due to a failure of properly managing the gut bacterial flora. Good bacteria in the intestine are needed, to produce two lectin-protective substances; *mucin and secretory IgA* (Bart Deplancke and H Rex Gaskins 2001).

Mucins have been called the *digestive gatekeepers*. They are a family of heavily sugar-coated proteins, secreted by mucous membrane as the principal components of mucus that coats many epithelial surfaces of the intestines and secreted also into fluids such as saliva.

Secretory IgA is an antibody produced by the immune system; they like to latch onto lectin and prevent them from causing damage.

When lectins travel through the intestines, if there is mucin, it will bind the lectin, neutralize it and safely escort it out of the body. When mucin and secretory IgA are missing, lectins will bind to intestinal cells instead (Jeffers F et al., 2010).

Mucins protect against yeast, bacteria and food sensitivities. Mucin contains the sugars that lectins like to stick to, including sialic acids (N-Acetylneuraminic acid).

Tomatoes contain *lycopene*, a powerful antioxidant. But tomatoes also contain *pan hemagglutinin*, a potentially harmful lectin. It lowers mucin, binds to blood cells and nerve tissues and interferes with gastrin (Robin Meywes).

If you have any health-related issues like allergies or hypothyroidism, it is very helpful to reduce your intake of problematic lectins. It's also very important to balance immunity by working on gut health. By consuming anti-microbial food and taking good quality probiotics you'll help stimulate adequate mucin and secretory IgA. (Nicholas J. Mantis, Ph.D. et al., 2011).

Bladderwrack is a seaweed found on the coasts of the North Sea, the western Baltic Sea, and the Atlantic and Pacific Oceans, also known by the common names black tang, rockweed, bladder fucus, sea oak, black tany, cut weed, dyers fucus, red fucus, and rock wrack.

Bladderwrack is rich in iodine, calcium, magnesium, potassium, sodium, sulfur, silicon and iron and high in some B-complex vitamins. It contains moderate amounts of phosphorus, selenium, manganese and zinc and small amounts of vitamins A, C, E and G. It also contains anti-sterility vitamin S, as well as vitamin K. It is rich in algin and mannitol, carotene and zeaxanthin with traces of bromine (Herb Wisdom).

Fucose, a sugar found in Bladderwack, not to be confused with fructose, is capable of binding to lectins.

This function may contribute to the prevention of Hashimoto Thyroiditis and its many complications.

Okra is a nutritional powerhouse used throughout history for both medicinal and culinary purposes. Okra rich content of nutrients includes vitamins and minerals, vitamins A, B, C, E, and K, as well as calcium, iron, magnesium, potassium, and zinc. Furthermore, okra contains high levels of mucilaginous fiber (Nutrition and you).

The mucilaginous and rich fiber content in okra cases helps enhance stool mass, binds poisons, eases digestion, relieves stomach ulcers, lubricates and cleans the intestines with its insoluble fibers.

The high vitamin C content can stimulate the immune system to create white blood cells, which can combat the other foreign pathogens and materials in the body that can weaken the immune system (Mike Barrett)

Myricetin is a flavonoid in okra also found in blueberries, garbanzo beans, turnips and chia seeds, among other foods, was isolated and dispensed to rats, which responded with increased sugar absorption in their muscles, consequently lowering their blood sugar (Liu IM et al., 2005).

Just a word of caution. Okra has high levels of oxalates. Oxalates bind to existing kidney and gallstones and cause them to grow and may worsen this condition. Remember, everything should be consumed in moderation.

D-mannose is a common binding sugar for lectins. It is capable of binding with the lectins and micro-organism in grains and other foods. D-mannose blocks the lectins in beans, peas, lentils and other legumes and prevents them from breaching the intestinal wall.

Mannose is not an essential nutrient; it can be produced in the human body from glucose or converted back into glucose. In addition, it occurs naturally in the cells lining the epithelial tract, the sugar D-mannose is also found in relatively large quantities in fruit such as peaches, pineapple, apples, oranges, and certain berries, like cranberries and blueberries (Breaking the vicious cycle).

Sodium alginate is a soluble fiber derived from seaweed and is resistant to digestion. It is fermented in part by the colonic bacteria to a highly beneficial short-chain fatty acid including butyrate, which is a favorite food for the colonic epithelial cells that use these fatty acids for energy.

Sodium alginate is also used for detoxification. Sodium alginate reacts with gastric acids to form a viscous gel called the alginate raft. This alginate raft surrounds lectins after they have attached to sugars, to rapidly eliminate them from the body. It also prevents acid reflux and esophageal burning (Mandel KG et al., 2000; Anderson DM et al., 1991).

L-Glutamine, the most abundant amino acid in blood, plays a vital role in the maintenance of mucosal integrity. Glutamine has traditionally been termed a non-essential amino acid, is now considered a conditionally essential amino acid. Its consumption in small bowel mucosa exceeds the rate of production during disease. In the small bowel mucosa, the amino acid L-glutamine is the principal source of energy both for maintaining and repairing intestinal mucous cells (Radha Krishna Rao and Geetha Samak 2011).

The foods with the most L-glutamine include bone broth, grass-fed beef, spirulina, Chinese cabbage, cottage cheese, asparagus, broccoli raab, wild caught fish (Cod, Tuna, and Salmon), venison, and turkey.

THE EPITHELIUM

The epithelium is one of the four basic types of animal tissue. The other three types are connective tissue, muscle tissue, and nervous tissue. Epithelial tissues line the cavities and surfaces of blood vessels and organs throughout the body. The *intestinal epithelium* is the layer of cells that forms the Luminal surface or lining of both the small and large *intestine* of the *gastrointestinal* tract (Wikipedia intestinal epithelium).

A key function of the intestine, besides absorption of nutrients, water, and electrolytes homeostasis, is to regulate the traffic of environmental antigens across the mucosal barrier. The tight intestinal junctions serve to ensure the optimal absorption and transport of nutrients and to control the balance between tolerance for self and immunity to non-self-antigens. To meet these diverse physiological challenges, the intestinal epithelial tight junctions must be modified rapidly and in a coordinated fashion by the regulatory systems (Alessio Fasano).

In the year 2000, researchers at the University of Maryland School of Medicine led by Dr. Fasano, discovered within the intestinal walls, this mysterious human protein called zonulin; the only human protein that so far can regulate the permeability of the intestine.

Increased intestinal permeability has been implicated in a range of autoimmune conditions including coeliac disease, type 1 diabetes, rheumatoid arthritis, and multiple sclerosis. In the presence of zonulin, the normally tight junctions between the intestinal cells remain open, creating bowel leakiness (GIOVANNI BARBARA 2015).

The experts tell us that monkeys and chimpanzees do not produce zonulin, and they rarely, if ever, develop autoimmune disorders. Human beings suffer from more than 70 different kinds of such conditions. It is believed that zonulin is the protein responsible for this difference between the species (News medical life science 2008).

Zonulin is the only known physiologic modulator of intercellular tight junction known to us so far (Carroccio et al. 2006).

Scientists found that intestinal bacterial infections and lectins trigger epithelial cells to release zonulin, initiating intestinal permeability, thereby enabling the passage of gliadin and other dietary and microbial antigens into the blood, which by interacting with the immune system give rise to inflammation. This vicious cycle is created and perpetuated due to the persistent presence of pro-inflammatory lectins (Drago S et al., 2006).

Dr. Fasano's group published a study showing that bacteria such as *E. coli, shigella* and *Salmonella* stimulate zonulin production in intestinal tissue, enhancing the ability of zonulin to create bowel leak (El Asmar R et al., 2002).

One of the most astounding findings of Dr. Fasano's work is that the gliadin-zonulin leak effect occurs not just in people with celiac disease or gluten-sensitivity; it occurs in everybody. Nobody is immune to this increased intestinal permeability. Not surprisingly, increased intestinal permeability has been associated with autoimmune diseases, such as type 1 diabetes, rheumatoid arthritis, and multiple sclerosis, and Hashimoto (Alessio Fasano).

Here is the science: When the epithelial cells are exposed to microbes, lectins or any other toxic chemicals, they release zonulin, which is designed to opens the tight juncture of the intestinal lining, allowing water to leak into the bowel, giving way to diarrhea. This is an adaptive response that develops in response to foreign invaders to flush them out of the body. If zonulin is present, these junctures will remain open. By ridding ourselves of the bacteria or offending lectin, the zonulin problem will disappear. (Food democracy 2013)

According to Chris Kresser M.S., LAc, doctor of functional and integrative medicine, Zonullin, the protein that protects the gut, is the same protein that protects the brain. So, if you have intestinal permeability, there is a good chance that you also have a compromised mental function (Chris Kresser).

The best approach to this dilemma is to increase the consumption of nutrients that will help to create the proper balance for the population of good bacteria in the gut to prevent both microorganisms and toxins like lectins from causing any problems in the intestines.

Bifidus **bacteria** for example has been proven to be a worthy anti-zonulin gastro-intestinal protector, virtually eliminating gluten's ability to cause damage (El Asmar R et al., 2002).

Short-chain fatty acids are produced by the friendly bacteria in your gut. In fact, they are the main source of nutrition for the cells in your colon. Short-chain fatty acids also play an important role in reducing the risk of inflammatory diseases like Hashimoto obesity, heart disease and other conditions (Kim YH et al., 2016).

Due to their anti-inflammatory and anti-cancer properties, it is likely that short-chain fatty acids have a wide range of beneficial effects on the body. One thing is certain: looking after your friendly gut bacteria can lead to a whole host of health benefits. The best way to feed the good bacteria in your gut is to eat a variety of fiber-rich foods, such as fruits, vegetables, and legumes, which are linked to an increase in short-chain fatty acids (Dr. Mary Jane Brown, RD).

Goji is a berry grows in the Himalayas and in the wild pristine low fertile soil of the Ningxia Province of China, has the highest concentration of antioxidants in the plant kingdom. One of the world's most powerful anti-aging food source, it has a complete spectrum of antioxidants, zeaxanthin, and carotenoids. It is loaded with omega-6, an excellent hormone regulator. It also boasts all the essential amino acids and twenty-one trace minerals, like iron, calcium, zinc, selenium, germanium, phosphorus, vitamins (C, B_1, B_2, B_6), and carotenoids, making Goji an antioxidant, antibacterial, anti-inflammatory, and immune system boosting.

Research has shown that Goji berries contain unique compounds known as *Lycium barbarum* polysaccharides, which have many immune-enhancing properties. These compounds enhance the body's ability to resist disease.

Goji berries help the immune system to distinguish more effectively between friend and foe. The fruit's polysaccharides provide cells with special sugars that support healthy immunity and enable cells to communicate more effectively with each other (Goji berries).

Author and pharmacist, Earl Mindell, calls Goji's polysaccharides "master molecules" because they command and control many of the body's most important biochemical defense systems.

Goji berries combination of fiber and polysaccharides support healthy immunity by naturally promoting the growth of healthy intestinal bacteria and protecting against unhealthy bacteria that cause disease (Adrian ASĂNICĂ).

Consumption of Goji berries increases energy level, athletic performance, quality of sleep, and ease of awakening, ability to focus on activities, mental acuity, calmness, and feelings of health, contentment, and happiness. Goji also significantly reduced fatigue and stress, and improved regularity of gastrointestinal function (Yin J, Xing H and Ye J. 2008).

Healing the gut may not be the only thing necessary to break free from Hashimoto thyroiditis, but it will keep us on course.

GRAVES' DISEASE

In Graves' disease, the keyword is *toxins*. A toxin is any substance produced by an organism that can cause disease when introduced into the body. Some healthy substances in excess are toxic to the body. These substances may include gliadin, histamine, and cortisol among many others.

Graves' disease is perpetrated by the presence of toxic substances, most of them coming from the food we consume, or from the environment. Once the body is completely detoxified, the disease ceases to exist. The body has a built-in mechanism design to eliminate toxins, it is accomplished is through the production of sweat. For sweating to take place, the body's temperature must increase. So, the immune system stimulates the thyroid gland to produce more thyroid hormones, which in turn increases metabolism and produces more heat in the body. Consequently, we begin to perspire. The more we sweat, the greater the amount of toxins that are excreted from the body.

Any prolonged or chronic exposure of the body to intoxicating substances stimulates the immune system into the production of thyroid-stimulating antibodies, which in turn forces the thyroid gland to produce more thyroid hormone. This leads to Graves' disease.

Chronic intoxication equals Graves' disease.

The immune system is very complex and often misunderstood, especially when dealing with health conditions like Graves' disease. However, from the very beginning, we must understand that this malady is treatable. The complexity is based on our ignorance about the disease. This leaves us with Synthroid or levothyroxine as the only solution.

According to WebMD (May 2015), Synthroid, the medication prescribed for Hashimoto and Graves' disease, is the number one prescribed medication in the United States. Alternative medicine is not totally in favor of using Synthroid, so it leans toward Armour thyroid; a natural product made from animal **thyroid** glands (usually a pig's).

We are fed the simplified hypothesis that the immune system somehow turns against the body and begins to destroy it by way of antibodies (Thyroid Foundation of Canada 2000). We have been mentally conditioned to believe that this disease comes about because of the existence of defective antibodies (American Thyroid Association 2016). However, to this day, science has not found any evidence to prove this theory as true (Mayo Clinic Staff 2014; Kronenberg et al. 2011; Wentz 2016).

When we closely analyze the limited information that is available to us about the workings of the immune system, we realize that when antibodies are directed at healthy cells of the body, they are not destructive, but regulating.

The peculiar thing about thyroid-stimulating immunoglobulins (which are produced by the immune system) is that they promote the growth of the thyroid gland, enabling it to increase production of the thyroid hormone. This effect of the antibodies on the thyroid gland seems uncharacteristic to us. So, our first impulse in treating Graves' disease is to focus all our efforts on correcting what we perceive to be a malfunction, when this immune system response is normal.

As a result, our attempt to fix the immune system is equivalent to chasing shadows in the dark. You can't straighten something that is not bent. No wonder Graves' disease is incurable because we are attempting to repair something that is not broken.

These thyroid-stimulating antibodies cause the thyroid gland to grow, which essentially is not bad. Under other circumstances, it would be necessary and beneficial. This feature of the immune system would come in useful if the thyroid gland were to become damaged or mutilated in any form as it happens in Hashimoto thyroiditis.

One of the roles of the immune system, though unexplored, is to exert a regulating influence upon the thyroid gland, causing it to produce more hormones if it sees the need, or to slow down the production of hormones if necessary. This is a wonderful faculty!

Based on this premise, we could conclude that even if the thyroid gland was damaged—as is the case of Hashimoto thyroiditis—the human immune system has the built-in mechanism to repair it and cause it to produce more hormones. The immune system could also cause the thyroid gland to produce fewer hormones.

Graves' disease is a normal immune response that has been prolonged due to the presence of too much intoxicating chemical in the body. Some of these toxins could be healthy nutrients of which we have eaten too much.

The problem that we face with the thyroid stimulating antibodies is that their production is chronic—they are being continually produced, and there is no stopping them. The obvious question now, is how do we halt the production of thyroid stimulating antibodies?

There are many factors that facilitate the development of Graves' disease. Some of them include: junk food (fast food and processed food), sugar, especially fructose, asbestos, lead, mercury, heavy metal, pesticides, air and water pollutants, tobacco, caffeine, cortisol in high doses, stress, alcohol, poor digestion, nutrition-depleted food, and consuming heated oil high in trans fatty acids and linoleic acids.

The cause of Graves' disease is a combination of chronic intoxication and an overabundance of substances like cortisol that suppresses the production of TSH. In rare cases, viral infections and pregnancy may also play a role.

High levels of cortisol interfere with the production of thyroid-stimulating hormones. In the absence of such hormones, a backup system comes into play in the form of thyroid-stimulating antibodies, produced by the immune system.

The pituitary gland is the regulator of the thyroid, when it fails to function as such, by default the responsibility falls on the immune system. Employing its thyroid-regulating ability, the immune system produces thyroid-stimulating immunoglobulins (also referred to as antibodies or autoantibodies) that can attach themselves to the thyrotropin receptors on the thyroid gland. The said receptors are usually reserved for thyroid-stimulating hormones proceeding from the pituitary gland.

These thyroid-stimulating antibodies have the same effect on the thyroid gland as the thyroid-stimulating hormones, which is to induce the gland to increase the production of thyroid hormone. As the levels of thyroid hormones increase in the blood, so does the body temperature, which produces perspiration. The secreted sweat carries toxins out of the body. This is a normal function of the immune system, meant to be a short-term solution—it is not an overreaction.

Sometimes the immune system produces these thyroid-stimulating antibodies almost nonstop, resulting in the overgrowth of the thyroid gland and overproduction of the thyroid hormone. When this happens, it is diagnosed as Graves' disease. Graves' disease is said to be the result of a malfunctioning or hyperactive immune system. However, just as is the case with Hashimoto, the proper wording should be an *over-stimulated* or a *hyper-stimulated* immune system.

Keep in mind that this situation is the result of a short supply of TSH. Once the TSH levels are normalized, the immune system will cease the production of TSI (thyroid stimulating immunoglobulin).

The immune system is a victim of *hyper-stimulation* if our natural impulse is to focus all our attention on fixing the immune system; we end up like a dog chasing its own tail. There is no catching it.

May I submit for your consideration the concept that Graves' disease is *not* the result of an overactive immune system, but that of a natural reaction of the immune system to an over-intoxicated body?

To reverse this disease, our attention must be drawn to a few main suspects. We mentioned toxins before; its partners in crime are either an overabundance of cortisol, histamine, or gliadin. Let us explore the existing relationship between Graves' disease, the immune system, toxins, and cortisol?

The immune system may be battling bacteria, parasites, viruses, allergens, and toxins all at the same time. Graves' disease develops when toxins become enemy number one. Under normal circumstances, our bodies should never become over-intoxicated, but in the case that it does happen, the immune system goes into action to rid the body of this unwanted guest—mainly by increasing body temperature.

When the production of thyroid-stimulating hormones is compromised—as it happens when there are elevated cortisol levels and a high concentration of inflammatory chemicals—then the immune system steps in to fill the gap (Briden 2013; Ruscio 2016). This should only be a short-term measure, just an emergency maneuver.

Now, let us put it into perspective; suppose that the body is constantly being assaulted by elevated levels of toxins. The immune system then finds itself locked into a detoxifying process gone chronic.

If during this confrontation against chronic intoxication, the body is assaulted by a suppressing agent like cortisol, the first thing that happens is the decrease in production of TSH by the pituitary gland. In the absence of an adequate supply of TSH, the immune system must take up the slack in order to keep the thyroid gland working. Cortisol also suppresses the T cells of the immune system, leaving them virtually paralyzed while it enhances the B cells, making them stronger and more active.

Under these circumstances, the size of the thyroid gland increases due to higher production of thyroid-stimulating antibodies. This is the reason why autoimmune disorders such as Graves' disease become noticeable just after we have undergone a stressful situation. Stress is the number one immune system suppressor by the production of cortisol.

Histamine tends to have that same effect as cortisol on the immune system and lectins are among the most toxic agents to the human body.

Suppose a woman becomes pregnant. Her body naturally shifts to a T_h2-dominant immune system, meaning her body's B cells are more active than the T cells. Let us then assume that a marital breakdown or another stressful situation develops. It drags on for many months and is highly emotionally stressful.

During those months of stress, the body will be constantly producing cortisol. Cortisol enhances the production and activity of B cells. When this happens, the population of B cells increases dramatically, and with that, the production of thyroid-stimulating antibodies. So, the immune system continues to produce these thyroid-stimulating antibodies without the ability to stop.

It is like driving a car and, say, a bottle of water rolls under the brake pedal. Because of this mishap, you lose control of your car and are unable to stop it. Imagine the bottle of water as cortisol and the brake pedal as the immune system. By removing the bottle of water, you are now able to stop your car, and by removing excess cortisol, we would once more gain control over our health, the immune system will then be able to operate freely, and the pituitary gland will once again resume control of the thyroid gland.

Recovery from Graves' disease is virtually a two-step process.

- First, it is necessary to undergo a complete body detoxification and at the same time abstain from toxic substances in food and the environment. This would mean a balanced diet should be involved.

- Second, reduce the level of cortisol or histamine to a minimum. This will bring balance to the immune system. Liberating it to resume operation free of restraints and bringing an immediate end to the production of antibodies.

The normal levels of TSH will also return. In time, the thyroid-stimulating antibodies will die off and the gland will resume normal operation.

To recover from Graves' disease, you must address the stressors in your life and sugar consumption. This pair may be responsible for the elevated cortisol levels. Keep a close eye also on allergy-causing substances; they will keep histamine levels soaring.

Lifestyle changes would not be too different from that of someone afflicted with Hashimoto thyroiditis. The only exception is that, in the case of Graves' disease, foods that should be part of your diet are those that are called goitrogens. That list includes soy and its related products, cauliflower, cabbage, radish, Brussels sprout, broccoli, kale, millet, cassava, pears, strawberries, and peaches. These foods contain substances that are contributors to slowing down the production of the thyroid hormone.

Overcoming Graves' disease is much easier if we incorporate super foods into our diet. The regular food that we consume does not have all the nutrients necessary to promote good health. Super-foods are nutrient dense. Most of them are organic, and they have the necessary elements in the proper ratio to promote healing. If they do not form part of your diet, you will find it difficult to recover because the body will be nutrient deprived.

Nutrients found in food can help us to manage this autoimmune disease and return the thyroid back to normal function (Michael Edwards).

Green tea could be your best friend in your fight against Graves' disease. It has antiviral, anti-inflammatory, and anti-cavity properties. Green tea contains powerful antioxidants that help to prevent cell damage. Green tea also suppresses both the production of thyroid hormone and thyroid-stimulating antibodies. This makes it a good candidate to help Graves' disease victims recover faster.

In that regard, there are many studies focusing on the conditions that favor immune system modulation. In this study published on PubMed, it was determined that the CD24 gene, if suppressed, could slow the activity of the immune system (PubMed.gov 2009)

CD24 is a protein-coding gene in humans. It helps to regulate cellular growth and differentiation. (NCBI 2016)

Cellular differentiation is the process by which a cell becomes specialized to perform a specific function. In this case, the cells that express the CD24 gene, become an antibody-producing cell. CD24 is expressed on the surface of B cells.

Green tea and **curcumin** suppress the expression of the CD24 gene on macrophage, neutrophils and the antibody-producing B cells. This contributes to the slowing of the thyroid autoimmune attacks on the thyroid cells. (Xiaohua Pan et al., 2015).

By limiting the expression of the CD24 gene, we can minimize the severity of this autoimmune condition and eventually send it into remission.

The natural supplement Curcumin, in a dose-dependent manner, has been shown to reduce the expression of CD24 (Hindawi Publishing Corporation) Curcumin is the yellow pigment associated with the curry spice, turmeric and to a lesser extent, Ginger.

Curcumin is an effective, inexpensive, and relatively safe polyphenolic compound isolated from the rhizome of the plant Curcuma longa that has traditionally been used for pain and wound-healing. Recent studies have shown that curcumin improves multiple sclerosis, rheumatoid arthritis, psoriasis, and inflammatory bowel disease in human or animal models. (Bright).

Curcumin along with green tea deliver a powerful one two punches against Graves' disease, because of their ability to limit the number and activity of immune system cells that are involved in the disease.

Many studies have demonstrated that Green tea inhibits the production of T3 and T4 hormones, and an increase in thyroid stimulating hormone production. (Israel today 2007)

In one study, the researchers noted a remarkable decrease in T3 and T4 thyroid hormone concentrations, in response to high doses of green tea (doses as high as 10, 20, and 30 mg/kg body weight). They also noted a significant rise in thyroid stimulating hormone (TSH) in response to a drop in thyroid hormone (T4) levels. (Suppversity-Nutrition and exercise science for everyone).

This is something good. ExcessT3 and T4 interfere in the regenerative process of the thyroid gland.

(Proceedings of the national academy of science of the United States of America) (Google search) (Wiley Online Library)

Anything that could decrease production of T3 or T4 is good for Graves' disease victims. The increase in TSH means that the pituitary gland is once again taking over the management of the thyroid gland which during the disease was under the management of the immune system. This will prevent the thyroid from being stimulated by thyroid stimulating antibodies.

Another reason for Green benefit for Graves' disease victims is due to its phenomenal efficiency in absorbing fluoride from the environment. The older the leaf, the higher the fluoride content.

Fluoride in Green tea leaf rose dramatically over the last 20 years due to industrial contamination. Recent analyses have revealed a fluoride content of 22.2 mg per tea-bag or cup in Chinese green tea, and 17.25 mg of soluble fluoride ions per tea-bag or cup in black tea. Aluminum content was also high—over 8 mg.

Mature leaves can contain ten to twenty times more fluoride than young leaves of the same plant. Green tea extract used in these studies are made from older and more mature leaves.

Young leaves are the best quality; they contain very little, if any, fluoride. So, I would suggest using only the Matcha brand of green tea, which is made from young leaves. (Thyroid U K Better thyroid health)

If the fires of Graves' disease are raging in your body, Green tea along with Ashwagandha, Rhodiola, curcumin and astragalos could be your best nutritional friends in modulating the immune system. Consider making these herbs a regular part of your life.

Astragalus is another powerful, liver-detoxifying agent that is well worth mentioning. It is an immune system booster that especially enhances T cells function, establishing balance in the system. Astragalus is of great benefit to those who suffer from Graves' disease because it promotes thyroid health.

Astragalus is known as the anti-aging herb. Its polysaccharides, beta-sitosterol, flavonoids, and trace minerals (especially selenium) protect the body from bacteria, virus, and free radicals. The calycosin and astragaloside compound in that it helps to reduce the amount of nitric oxide released from cells, causing inflammation to decline.

Astragalus boosts the immune system by increasing the rate of replication of immune cells called macrophages. Due to this fact, many health professionals advise against taking Astragalus if you have Hashimoto because a boosted immune system could cause more damage to the thyroid gland when in attack mode. However, for hyperthyroism, it is great (University of Maryland Medical Center 2016).

Its daily recommended allowance is 200 to 500 mg (Bechtel 2012; Group 2015; DrWeil.com 2015). I used the powdered root, two teaspoons of it daily.

According to the National Center for Complementary and Alternative Medicine, Astragalus can interfere with medications that suppress the immune system, blood sugar, and blood pressure—which may be fatal. Talk to your physician prior to taking Astragalus (Wood-Moen 2011).

Rhodiola grows in the arctic regions of Asia and Europe, and the best quality is said to be Siberian grown. Rhodiola enhances the immunity in three different ways:

1. By stimulating "natural killer cells" (NK cell) in the stomach and spleen. NK-cells, seek out and destroy the infected cells in your body. This effect contributes to the regeneration of the thyroid gland.
2. By improving your T-cell immunity. It maximizes your body's resistance to the toxins that accumulate during an infection.
3. By its ability to reduce cortisol. Cortisol suppresses the immune system. (J Med Food 2010) (Underground health reporter)

Rhodiola is not a herb to take while with hypothyroidism. It will cause your condition to deteriorate because it lowers cortisol levels. Low cortisol levels are characteristic of Hashimoto.

Graves' disease is characteristic of high levels of cortisol, which means that the adaptogen herb Rhodiola is an excellent addition to your anti-Graves arsenal. One of its special attributes is that it lowers cortisol levels and stabilizes thyroid hormone production.

The recommended daily allowance for this anti-stress and anti-inflammatory herb is between 200 to 600 mg daily (Merely Me 2010).

Vitamin E: deficiency of this vitamin encourages the thyroid gland to secrete too much hormone, as well as too little TSH by the pituitary gland.

A higher intake of vitamin E is often needed by people with an overactive thyroid to counteract the large amounts of the vitamin depleted from the system.

Vitamin E promotes selenium metabolism. Therefore, taking vitamin E without selenium will quickly deplete the body's store of the mineral and lead to hyperthyroidism or hypothyroidism.

In fact, vitamin E deficiency affects the thyroid more severely when it is accompanied by selenium deficiency.

B6 (Pyridoxine) deficiencies can lead to low serotonin levels and sleep problems, muscle weakness, and make your immune system more prone to attack your thyroid gland. Without this vitamin, the thyroid cannot use its iodine raw material efficiently to make the hormones. This vitamin is needed even more by those who have an overactive thyroid.

It has been found that when people with an overactive thyroid take vitamin D, it counteracts the usual rapid excretion of calcium, and osteoporosis can be avoided. Health Canada recommends that men and women over the age of 50 take a daily supplement of 400 IU. You can get vitamin D from fortified milk, yogurt, and orange juice.

Vitamin C: Long standing deficiency of vitamin C causes the thyroid gland to secrete too much hormone. People with an overactive thyroid need extra Vitamin C as this is drained from the tissues in their bodies.

A study published in the "American Journal of Clinical Nutrition," vol 40 in 1984 showed that zinc levels were higher by a significant amount in those patients with hypothyroidism, and significantly lower in those with hyperthyroidism. The same study showed that copper was lower in patients with hypothyroidism, and higher in those with hyperthyroidism (Jabar et al.)

If Graves' disease is your affliction, this could be your starting point in your journey back to normal, which could take anywhere from six to eighteen months. It is much easier said than done, so patience will be one of your biggest assets on this journey.

Once the body is maintained in a detoxified state and all restrictions of the immune system have been removed, the body will return to normal operation (National Center for Complementary and Integrative Health 2016).

Glutathione is the most important antioxidant in the body, and it has a wide range of scientifically proven health effects. It is a sticky molecule that acts like a magnet attracting all the free radical, toxins and heavy metal in the body to stick onto it.

Glutathione is a master detoxifier responsible for the health and well-being of every cell in the body. It is the secret to gracefully aging, good quality of life, improved autoimmune function, DNA health, energy production, reduction of inflammation, and as an effective treatment for everything from autism to Alzheimer's disease (Mark Hyman).

Glutathione keeps the liver healthy by eliminating free radicals from the body and in reducing and repairing the damage they caused. It also inhibits the production of most inflammatory cytokines (Pietro Ghezzi)

Dr. Joseph Mercola describe free radicals as "reactive particles that bounce all around the cell, damaging everything they touch." Most are by-products of the process of metabolism, but they also originate from exposure to toxins, radiation, and toxic metals.

Glutathione also protects the intestinal mucosa and gut wall from becoming weak which could lead to leaky gut (Johannes et al.)

Unfortunately, poor diet, pollution, toxins, medications, stress, trauma, old age, sugar, infections and radiation all deplete glutathione, leaving you susceptible to unrestrained cell disintegration and the many diseases that we suffer as a result (Kenichi Kitani)

You can enhance internal glutathione production by increasing factors that boost it; the amino acids L-cysteine, glycine, and L-glutamate; vitamins B6, B12, vitamins C, and E (Masahiro et al.).

You can boost your glutathione directly by eating protein-rich foods like fruits and vegetables. Glutathione is sold in dietary supplement form as well. Many people say supplemental glutathione doesn't make it through your digestive tract, but studies in both humans and rodents show it is efficiently absorbed across the intestinal epithelium (Richie et al.)

Thyroid Regeneration

The medical community identifies six body tissues as having regenerative capacity. They are the liver, nerves, beta cells or insulin-producing cell, hormones, cardiac cells and joint and spine cartilage. (GreenMedinfo)

Although the thyroid gland has the regenerative properties to grow when stimulated, it is not deemed to be a regenerating organ. It is looked upon as a dormant organ. (Cancer Survivors Network 2011; Wentz 2016; Hanson et al. 2012; Kronenberg et al. 2011).

The cells of the thyroid gland divide approximately five times during adult life. (Endocrine Society) Despite this, it maintains the ability to grow through two distinct processes at the same time: hypertrophy and hyperplasia.

- **Hypertrophy** is the increase in the volume of an organ or tissue due to the enlargement of the cells of which it is composed. (Springer Link)
- **Hyperplasia** is the increase in the number of cells while the organ remains approximately the same size. (PMC frontier in endocrinology)

Most physicians and endocrinologists believe in Hashimoto thyroiditis, the hypothyroid condition, is irreversible. However, this isn't true! It has been demonstrated in various studies, which after the inflammation dies down, thyroid function spontaneously returned in 20% of patients with Hashimoto.

These individuals will return to normal thyroid function, especially after thyroid hormone replacement has been withdrawn. (Mary Ann Liebert, Inc. Publishing)

Several studies demonstrate the ability of the thyroid gland to regenerate and regain its normal function, even after almost complete destruction or thyroidectomy of the gland.

Regeneration of the thyroid would be a common occurrence if victims of Hashimoto did not rely so fully, on Synthetic or animal thyroid hormone replacement. The use of these supplements interferes with the regenerating ability of the thyroid because they neutralize the stimulating process of the TSH. The thyroid gland will regain normal function faster if we avoid thyroid hormone supplements and permit the natural process of stimulation of the thyroid to run its course.

Nevertheless, being aware that the regeneration process of the thyroid after the disease has gone into remission is slow, if you want to use a thyroid hormone supplement, do it. However, limit yourself to only a partial dose, this will leave room for the thyroid gland to be stimulated by TSH, to make up the difference.

TSH plays a key role in the regenerating process of the thyroid. (Endocrine Society) Because, the thyroid gland must be stimulated by Thyroid stimulating hormone or Thyroid stimulating antibodies, for it to regenerate.

Graves' disease victims do not have a problem in this respect. Because in Graves' disease, the immune system produces autoantibodies that stimulate the thyroid gland into growth (Dayan and Saravanan 2001).

Graves' disease develops when the normal autoimmunity of the body spirals out of control. Once the immune system returns to normal, these same autoantibodies will cause the thyroid gland to generate new cells and produce more hormones. The body naturally produces these thyroid-stimulating antibodies. The process is called *low-level autoimmunity*, which is normal (Mandal 2014; Agapov et al. 2012; Wadi 2014; Hecht 2008).

Even with Hashimoto's sufferers: they develop a goiter, which is proof of the growing ability of the thyroid gland. A goiter is more a normal response of the thyroid than a disease symptom. Unfortunately, most of us only experience it during disease. So, we have come to mistakenly associate goiter with the abnormal.

After Hashimoto goes into remission, it is possible to have the gland regrow and resume normal operation, (Thyroid is the latest success in regenerative medicine 2016).

Nutrients found in food can help us to manage this autoimmune disease and return the thyroid back to normal function (Michael Edwards).

In that regard, there are many studies focusing on the conditions that favor thyroid regeneration. In this study published on PubMed, it was determined that the regeneration of the thyroid gland is faster when low levels of CD24 prevail (PubMed.gov 2009).

CD24 is a protein-coding gene in humans. It helps to regulate cellular growth and differentiation. (NCBI 2016)

Cellular differentiation is the process by which a cell becomes specialized to perform a specific function. In this case, the cells that express the CD24 gene, become an antibody-producing cell. CD24 is expressed on the surface of B cells.

By limiting the expression of the CD24 gene, we can minimize the severity of this autoimmune condition and eventually send it into remission.

The natural supplement Curcumin, in a dose-dependent manner, has been shown to reduce the expression of CD24 (Hindawi Publishing Corporation) Curcumin is the yellow pigment associated with the curry spice, turmeric and to a lesser extent, Ginger.

Curcumin is an effective, inexpensive, and relatively safe polyphenolic compound isolated from the rhizome of the plant Curcuma longa that has traditionally been used for pain and wound-healing. Recent studies have shown that curcumin improves multiple sclerosis, rheumatoid arthritis, psoriasis, and inflammatory bowel disease in human or animal models. (Bright)

Curcumin is the main active ingredient in turmeric. However, the curcumin content of turmeric is not that high… it's around 3% by weight.

Curcumin has powerful anti-inflammatory benefits that can be helpful in autoimmune conditions. Specifically, by down-regulating Th-1 cytokines, which may be overactive in Hashimoto's. Curcumin also neutralizes free radicals on its own and stimulates the production of the body's own antioxidant enzymes. (Dr. Izabella Wentz Pharm D 2015)

In an animal model of hypothyroidism, turmeric extract treatment was found to reduce atrophy (reduction in size) of thyroid glands and prevents reduction of thyroid hormone levels. It was also found that turmeric helps stimulate thyroid hormone production in hypothyroidism and to alleviate high levels of cholesterol caused by hypothyroidism (Deshpande et al.).

A study published in the Indian Journal of Endocrinology and Metabolism investigated the role of dietary turmeric in development of goitre. A total of 2335 residents of Pak Pattan, Punjab, Pakistan were interviewed. The population had a high prevalence of hyperthyroidism and endemic goitre. Interestingly, goitre was less common in those individuals who consumed milk, ghee, spices, chillies and turmeric. The researchers emphasized that turmeric use was associated with reduced goitre development and recommended inclusion of turmeric in diet in cases of goitre (Jawa a et al., 2015)

Curcumin has years of traditional use and some preliminary convincing research. However, there is no standard dosage. Ask your health care provider for advice.

Curcumin, however, is poorly absorbed into the bloodstream, thus it should be enhanced with other agents such as black pepper extract, called piperine, which enhances the absorption of curcumin by 2000%.

Most of the studies on this herb have been conducted using turmeric extract that contains mostly curcumin, with dosages usually exceeding 1 gram per day. It would be very difficult to reach these levels just using the turmeric spice in your foods. Therefore, if you want to experience the full effect of curcumin, you need to consider buying the curcumin extract, not turmeric powder.

Find a curcumin supplement that has been enhanced with Bioperine. Bioperine or piperine, is an extract of black pepper. (Authority on nutrition)

Dietary turmeric can benefit in reducing risk of thyroid disorders as well as benefit in treatment. According to the University of Maryland Medical Center, Turmeric can be taken with a supplement called bromelain to help reduce inflammation, typically taken between meals, 500 mg three times daily, Standardized powder (curcumin): 400 to 600 mg, 3 times per day

- Fluid extract (1:1) 30 to 90 drops a day
- Tincture (1:2): 15 to 30 drops, 4 times per day (University of Maryland medical center)

Green tea suppresses the expression of the CD24 gene on macrophage, neutrophils and the antibody-producing B cells. This contributes to the slowing of the thyroid autoimmune attacks on the thyroid cells. (Xiaohua Pan et al., 2015).

Green tea initially also inhibits thyroid hormone secretion, however, in so doing, it facilitates the production of TSH, which in turn, stimulates growth of the thyroid gland. Because of this growth, the levels of thyroid hormones will increase, compensating for the initial suppressing effect.

Because of the suppressing effects Green tea exerts on the thyroid gland, it should only be used as a short-term solution, for not more than 4 to six weeks at the beginning of your treatment of the disease; just enough time to blunt the autoimmune attacks on the thyroid gland.

After that initial period, drop the Green tea and continue only with curcumin and other nutrients.

Remember, Green tea could help in halting the autoimmune attack, so, only use it for that purpose. Using it after that will only make you feel increasingly weaker.

The role of "Thyroid Stimulating Hormone in thyroid regeneration:" Thyroid Stimulating Hormone (TSH) is produced by the pituitary gland with the purpose of stimulating the thyroid gland into secretion of thyroid hormone (T4). However, there is a secondary purpose usually viewed as an undesirable attribute. When the thyroid gland is sluggish, the TSH will stimulate it into growth to meet the required demand for thyroid hormone; this growth is called a goiter.

After the autoimmune attacks on the thyroid gland stop, the thyroid remains mutilated. For it to produce adequate amount of thyroid hormone, it must generate new cells to replace the ones that were destroyed. Enlargement of the thyroid gland is what you need at this point. TSH does that. We need to learn to appreciate this attribute of the thyroid gland and learn the principle involved in stimulating it into action so that we could regain a normal functioning thyroid gland.

Resveratrol is a polyphenol that is found in fruits. It possesses medicinal properties that are beneficial in various diseases. Scientists have discovered that Resveratrol enhances the growth of the thyroid gland by stimulating the pituitary gland to secrete thyroid stimulating hormone (Giuliani et al.). Resveratrol also influences thyroid function by enhancing iodide trapping. Put Resveratrol on your "to eat" list.

Along with Resveratrol, the body requires adequate amounts of protein, magnesium, and vitamin B12 in the diet to produce TSH.

According to an April 2009 study published in the journal *Clinical Nutrition*, the hypothalamus requires zinc to make the hormone it uses to signal the pituitary gland to make TSH to activate the thyroid. Deficiency of zinc can result in hypothyroidism. Conversely, hypothyroidism can result in zinc deficiency. The hair loss attributed to hypothyroidism may not improve even if you are on thyroxine unless zinc supplements are added. (Ambooken et. Al., 2013)

Zinc is required to produce T4 and for the conversion to the active form of thyroid hormone known as T3. These T3s enter your cells and fire up the energy-producing parts of your cell known as mitochondria. Zinc is required for T3 receptors in your cells to work. So, even if you have enough T3, it won't work optimally if you are deficient in Zinc.

Zinc deficiency is characterized by poor wound healing, loss of appetite, weight loss and white marks on the fingernails (David Gutrierrez, Natural News).

If you are Zinc-deficient taking 30-60mg of Zinc a day with food for 30 days and then retesting is recommended. It may take up to 60 days to replenish your Zinc levels. Make sure your Zinc supplement has a small amount of copper in it because taking Zinc will deplete your body of this important mineral (DR. Nikolas Hedberg, D.C., D.A.B.I)

The Best Foods for Natural Zinc Supplementation: Oysters, Soy protein, Liver, Veal, Beans, Elk, Lobster, Beef, Lamb, Endive

Copper and zinc have a complex relationship when it comes to your body's health and proper thyroid performance. You need both copper and zinc in sufficient levels to prevent and correct thyroid disorders (Dr. Atkins).

Copper stimulates the thyroid gland, and at the same time, protects the body against too much thyroxine in the blood. A study published in the "American Journal of Clinical Nutrition," vol 40 in 1984 showed that copper was lower in patients with hypothyroidism, (Jabar et al.)

Safe levels of copper supplements are between 1.5 and 3 mg per day for adults. Children should not take more than 2.5 mg per day. The Best Foods for Natural Copper Supplementation: liver, oysters, Sesame seeds, cocoa powder and unsweetened chocolate, nuts, lobster, sunflower seeds, tomatoes, pumpkin seeds.

Melatonin is secreted by the pineal gland during the night and benefits us in multiple ways including the regulation of circadian and seasonal rhythms as antioxidant and as anti-inflammatory. Melatonin therapy has been investigated in several animal models of autoimmune disease where it has proven to have a beneficial effect in a good deal of autoimmune health related conditions except rheumatoid arthritis. (Gu-Jiun Lin et al.).

A team of researchers led by Sakamoto S. conducted a study in which the results demonstrated that melatonin has a direct effect on thyroid hormone by stimulating the accumulation of TSH (Sakamoto et al.).

In another study, 3 mg of melatonin were given to perimenopausal and menopausal women for six months, which showed a remarkable and highly significant improvement of thyroid function and increased level of thyroid hormone. So, in your treatment for Hashimoto Thyroiditis, I suggest you seriously consider the impact that melatonin could have on the regeneration of your thyroid (Bellipanni et al.).

Protein

Proteins are essential nutrients found throughout the body. We are made up of about ten-thousand proteins, most of which are fabricated by the body. Every day we need to be provided with nine essential amino acids, these are proteins that the body cannot manufacture so they must be provided in the food we eat. Of these nine, the body then makes thirteen more, bringing the number up to twenty-two.

Using these twenty-two amino acids, the body synthesizes all the protein that is needed for its proper functioning.

Of interest to us, are the protein asparagine, leucine and tyrosine. These proteins are vital for producing thyroid hormone and getting it into the cells. Without them, the thyroid hormone is left stranded; the cells then starve and become weak (Tom Brimeyer).

Asparagine is an amino acid that makes up thyroid stimulating hormone (TSH). This protein deficiency is common and can lead to hypothyroidism.

Asparagine is a non-essential amino acid manufactured from other amino acids in the liver. When the body is low on asparagine, we could get it from poultry, dairy, eggs, fish, lactalbumin, legumes, meat, nuts, seafood, seeds, soy, whey, whole grains, and beef.

Leucine is an essential branched-chain amino acid used in the liver, fat tissue, and muscle tissue. Leucine builds and repairs your body, especially muscle tissue and helps prevent the deterioration of muscle with that comes with age. Leucine is required to power up the thyroid hormone so that your metabolism function at a high level.

High leucine foods include cheese, soybeans, beef, chicken, pork, nuts, seeds, fish, seafood, and beans. The recommended daily intake for leucine is 39mg per kilogram of body weight, or 17.7mg per pound. A person weighing 70kg (~154 pounds) should consume around 2730mg of leucine per day.

Tyrosine is a non-essential amino acid that is indispensable for making neurotransmitters in brain. Tyrosine also helps to regulate a variety of hormones that are produced by the thyroid, adrenal gland, and pituitary gland. It is also a precursor to thyroid hormone.

Tyrosine is found in soy products, chicken, turkey, fish, peanuts, almonds, avocados, bananas, milk, cheese, yogurt, cottage cheese, lima beans, pumpkin seeds, and sesame seeds."

The best way to get more protein is to make sure you're eating enough protein rich foods

Rich sources of amino acids are: chicken, turkey, fish, pork, beef, dairy products, lamb, and eggs.

It has been suggested that the average woman needs about forty-six grams of protein daily, while an average male should consume fifty-six grams (Nutritional-Supplements-Health-Guide.com 2016; Appleby 2016).

An adequate daily supply of amino acids is required for everyone, but especially for those seeking to recover from Hashimoto thyroiditis. For those of us who do not consume animal products, there are some excellent sources of amino acids (maybe even better ones than what we get from animals) available at health food stores.

Magnesium: According to the National Institute of Health, magnesium helps develops bones, regulate blood sugar, improves mood, controls the nervous system, keeps the heart regulated, and can help lessen PMS symptoms.

Many adults are magnesium deficient, thanks to the reduction in minerals in the average person diet.

A lack of magnesium causes a variety of symptoms, but one of the most common ones is improper thyroid function.

Magnesium stimulate the thyroid gland to produce more T4, but it simultaneously helps to changes T4 into T3. This is the reason why magnesium is so vital.

The National Institute of Health recommends that healthy adults consume about 400 mg of magnesium daily. Magnesium is present in many foods, including leafy vegetables, nuts, rice, meat, fish, pumpkin, bananas and whole grains.

Vitamin B12 is found in every cell of the body. It is required for cellular metabolism and energy production. B12 deficiencies are very common in people with an underactive thyroid or those with no thyroid. A serious lack of B12 can cause mental illness, neurological disorders, neuralgia, neuritis, bursitis, and can cause or worsen hypothyroidism.

Even though most people consume enough vitamin B12 in their diets, a deficiency occurs in many due to an inability to absorb the nutrient in the blood. This goes back to digestive health. The body cannot absorb and assimilate nutrients properly with a poorly functioning digestive system.

In addition, if the liver is not healthy, this radically inhibits the body's ability to utilize B12. Some doctors believe the normal range of B12 should be at least 500 - 1,300pg/ml (rather than 200 - 1,100).

Detrimental foods

Many plant foods contain naturally occurring chemicals which disrupt normal thyroid function, making it difficult for the thyroid to make enough thyroid hormone. Whenever this happens the thyroid gland grows, forming a goiter to do a better job (Creswell et al.).

The ability of the thyroid gland to enlarge is good, but only at the right time. After Hashimoto goes into remission, you will be left with a mutilated thyroid gland that must then generate new cells and grow to produce an adequate level of thyroid hormones. However, while the disease is still raging is not the time!

Substances that have this effect on the thyroid gland are called goitrogens

Goitrin is the most powerful plant goitrogen. This chemical can cause goiter even if there is plenty of iodine in the diet. It is found in cruciferous vegetables such as cabbage, brussels sprouts and rapeseed oil (Lüthy et al.).

Thiocyanates are sulfur-containing goitrogenic compounds that compete with iodine for entry into the thyroid gland. One way to deal with these chemical compounds is by supplementing the diet with iodine; the excess iodine will then crowd out the thiocyanate and win the competition.

Broccoli contains a substance called glucosinolate. Cassava and flaxseed have limarin. When the plant is cut, crushed, or chewed these substances turn into hydrocyanic acid (*cyanide*), which is very toxic, so the human body converts them into thiocyanate which is less toxic than cyanide and easier for the body to eliminate, but it does interfere with thyroid function (FAO).

Genestein, the soy flavonoid, reduces the activity of thyroid peroxidase, the enzyme required to insert iodine into thyroid hormone. Cooking does not destroy the goitrogenic activity of soy genestein, making it the strongest thyroid suppressor.

Apigenin is the most potent millet flavonoid. The other two are glucosylorientine and vitexin. These are on the same level with the goitrogen in soy in that cooking does not destroy these millet flavonoids.

Quercetin and its relatives interfere with thyroid hormone metabolism by reducing the activity of thyroperoxidase, and by reducing activity of hepatic deiodinase, a liver enzyme required to activate thyroid hormone. Quercetin is found in significant amounts in capers, cranberries, onions, green tea, broccoli, red wine, black currants, apples, grapes, blueberries, gingko biloba, and apricots (Greer MA)

Kaempferol found in significant amounts in green tea, capers, grapefruit, and endive. Kaempferol is closely related to quercetin and even more easily absorbed.

Rutin found in significant amounts in buckwheat, asparagus, citrus fruits, cranberries. Rutin is also a close relative of quercetin, but less well absorbed.

Boiling destroys up to 30 percent of the quercetin, kaempferol and rutin in food (Georgia Ede MD).

Moderate Thyroid Inhibitors are cruciferous vegetables: bok choy, broccoli, Brussels sprouts, cabbage, cauliflower, garden cress, kale, kohlrabi, mustard, mustard greens, radishes, rutabagas, turnips.

Mild Thyroid Inhibitors include: bamboo shoots, peaches, peanuts, cassava, flax, pears, pine nuts, radishes, spinach, strawberries, and sweet potatoes.

If you steam vegetables, it decreases goitrogen yield by about 30 percent, 70 percent remains in the food. Boil them for 1/2 hour, keep the water and 65 percent of the goitrogens are removed. If you throw away the water, about 90 percent of goitrogens are removed along with the nutrient. What then would be the point of eating nutrients that are vegetable deprived? (Meridian Health Clinic)

It has been said that fermenting or culturing these foods, reduces its goitrogenic effect. However, fermenting cabbage into sauerkraut increases the goitrogens that it contains.

For people with regular hypothyroidism, a small amount of goitrogenic food may not pose a problem. But If you have Hashimoto Thyroiditis or have only a partially functional thyroid and you have been a heavy consumer of cooked or raw goitrogens you should consider cutting back on the amount of these foods in your diet.

Look at it this way: Hashimoto Thyroiditis is a sickness in which your thyroid is been battered and mutilated every day by the immune system; the health of the thyroid is compromised. You do not have the good fortune of being able to eat goitrogens without running the risk of further affecting the thyroid negatively. If you are to recover, at some point you must stop consuming the goitrogen.

Try to find other foods to replace the nutrition you may be missing from these goitrogenic foods, at least until the damage to the gland has been repaired, and it is back to normal functioning. It boils down to whether you want to only survive with the disease or overcome it.

Mercury, Fluoride, Chlorine, Bromide, amiodarone, and Carbamazepine are chemical substances which can also have a goitrogenic effect on the thyroid function. Try to keep them away from you.

The Adrenals

The adrenal glands are located just above the kidneys, which are in the middle of your lower back area. You have one adrenal gland for each kidney. The right adrenal gland is triangular-shaped, and the left adrenal gland is shaped like a half-moon. They are approximately 2.5 inches long and 1 inch wide, and they have a yellowish color (Fawne Hansen).

Each adrenal gland is divided into an outer cortex and an inner medulla. They're involved in producing over 50 hormones that drive almost every bodily function.

The adrenals are of interest to us because of its relationship with the immune system. One of the principal hormones secrete by the adrenal is cortisol.

Chronic excessive levels of cortisol are seen in an autoimmune condition known as Cushing's syndrome. Chronically low and insufficient levels of cortisol are seen in another autoimmune condition called Addison's disease. So, whether the levels of cortisol are too high or too low; they both lead to autoimmune conditions.

When the adrenal glands function below the necessary level, it is most commonly associated with intense or prolonged stress, or after acute or chronic infections, especially respiratory infections such as influenza, bronchitis or pneumonia, it is referred to as Adrenal fatigue.

Adrenal fatigue is a relatively new term in the natural health world. It was proposed as a new condition by Dr. James L. Wilson a naturopath and chiropractor. He assumed that chronic stress over time could lead to an over production of cortisol in the bloodstream sometimes and under-production at other times.

Adrenal fatigue is a condition where your adrenal glands cannot keep up with the daily stress of life. When the adrenals stop producing hormones efficiently, every bodily function is affected, and adrenal hormone levels flow abnormally, giving way to symptoms that include autoimmune conditions (Allen V Jr).

Common symptoms of adrenal fatigue include severe tiredness, brain fog, decreased sex drive, hair loss, insulin resistance and others.

Stressful experiences, exposure to environmental toxins, pollution, financial hardship, bad relationships, work environment, consistent negative thinking, emotional trauma, lack of sleep, poor diet, food sensitivities, surgery, and reliance on stimulants are all contributors to adrenal fatigue (Duan et al.)

Wellness doctors and practitioners believe that prolonged, chronic stress can cause adrenal glands to become overloaded and ineffective in releasing cortisol.

Depression also plays a role in the development of adrenal fatigue. After a major depressive episode, cortisol responses do not easily readjust to normal levels and could contribute to the development of adrenal fatigue (Morris MC and Rao U).

Sleep is another important factor with the adrenals. Researchers at Brandeis University discovered that the *quality* could affect adrenal response more than the *quantity* of sleep (Bassett et al.).

Often, adrenal fatigue is characterized by an overabundance of cortisol. However, there comes a time when the adrenals are not able to produce enough cortisol to meet the body's daily demand; this is known as adrenal insufficiency.

One study shows that immune responses are limited in people suffering from adrenal insufficiency: they are physiologically incapable of responding to pathogens, like healthy individuals do (Geiger et al.).

To recover from adrenal fatigue or insufficiency is not easy. You may however, notice a difference in your overall well-being after just a few weeks of a healthier lifestyle.

It will take some time, an average of 6 months. However, it is scientifically proven that it's possible to improve adrenal function by practicing meditation or positive self-talk (Eagleson et al.)

To naturally fight adrenal fatigue, remove inflammatory foods from your diet, especially sugar and excess carbohydrates, and eat plenty of colorful, plant-based foods, free-range lean meats such as chicken or turkey, and lots of healthy fats.

One herb that has gained a reputation for strengthening the adrenals is Ashwagandha.

Ashwagandha is an adaptogen herb that has shown incredible results for lowering cortisol and balancing thyroid hormones. It helps the body to cope with stress. It boosts the immune system by increasing the white blood cell count. The herb is antibacterial, antioxidant, and anti-inflammatory.

If you want to look younger, restore your energy, and reverse disease then ashwagandha may be the herb you're looking for.

Ashwagandha has traditionally been used to strengthen the immune system after illness. Ashwagandha has also been proven effective in supporting adrenal function helping the overcome adrenal fatigue and chronic stress.

Medical studies have shown that ashwagandha improves cortisol levels, insulin sensitivity and naturally balances hormones.

Ashwagandha is considered by some health care providers as the number one herb for thyroid improvement although, the dynamics are not fully understood. One-half to one teaspoon of the herb is the recommended daily allowance (Kar and Panda 1998; Dr. Axe 2016).

NUTRITION

To overcome Hashimoto, you need to begin to think natural foods. Fruits, vegetables, grains, seeds, nuts, and some roots. These contain nutrients in the proper balance to keep the human body in good condition. The only processing, they require is that of digestion.

Hashimoto is a disease caused by nutrient imbalances. When the body has sufficient supply of nutrients, no invader could breach its defenses, which means that the first step back to the path of health, is to re-establish the delicate nutritional balance of essential nutrients, which are required for optimal health.

Essential nutrients (carbohydrates, proteins, fats, vitamins, water, and minerals), cannot be made by the body and must be provided in the diet (Amanda Hernandez).

To meet your quota of sufficient nutrients to beat this illness, you must up the ante with super-foods! They are jam-packed with nutrients. They will not all work for you, so you will need to engage in some trial and error. Some may taste more like medicine, but remember; we are not that healthy. If the food is going to reward you with healing, it will be worth getting used to the taste.

Although you may not be able to escape taking supplements, do not rely entirely on supplements. Nutrients like iodine, calcium, and vitamin D, vitamin A resveratrol and a few others may have to be supplemented, but try to keep supplementation to a minimum.

Let us now look at some of the essential nutrients and foods that I found to be effective in treating Hashimoto.

Water

There are many factors that contribute to the maintenance of optimal health, one of them is water. It is believed that if an adequate amount of water was to be maintained in our bodies, we would never become sick. On the other hand, the lack of water in our system will lead to dehydration and ultimately ill health (D'Anci et al. 2010).

The primary function of water is to hydrate the cells of our body. Its other important roles are cushioning the brain, lubricating the joints, transporting nutrients, taking waste away from cells, and regulating body temperature (European Hydration Institute 2016).

It has been drilled into our brain that to maintain hydration of the cells of the body, one needs to drink, on average, eight glasses of water daily. However, this depends on the height and weight of the individual (Gunnars 2016).

When I lived in Nicaragua, a tropical country, I experienced a lot of perspiration, even when inactive. I also was very physically active, so I needed more than ten glasses of water a day. However, when I moved back to Canada, where the temperature is much cooler than the tropics, I discovered that my body didn't need that much water anymore. Even six glasses of water in the middle of winter proved to be almost too much.

With Hashimoto disease, one needs to keep in touch with his or her body and take note how everything that one ingests is affecting it. For me, I did notice that ten glasses of water in Nicaragua were fine, but in Canada, I had to get up multiple times during the night to urinate. This wasn't good because it interfered with the quality of sleep that I was receiving. Waking up once a night was okay, but more than that left me tired the next day. So, I reduced the amount of water to six glasses a day, which worked much better.

One thing worth keeping in mind is that water and juice are not the same. There is a difference between pure water and altered water—whether it is lemonade, tea, coffee, sweetened beverages, juice—and mineralized or alkalized water.

When we ingest pure water, it goes directly to hydrate the cells of the body, not having to go through the digestive process. Recent studies show that water ingested on an empty stomach begins to enter the bloodstream within five minutes (Häussinger 1996). On the other hand, once we change the composition of water by adding a chemical component—be it minerals, vitamins, sugar or anything else—that water instead must go through the digestive process first in order to separate the water from the nutrients and other chemicals that we have mixed into it.

The latter end of the digestive process goes as follows: the nutrients, along with water that is absorbed from the intestines, enter the bloodstream and go directly to the liver, which purifies it, removing all the toxic materials. This purified blood then is transported to the kidneys, whose job is to remove all the extra material from the blood. As blood passes through the kidneys, they remove everything that is in excess at that moment, so all this excess water that is in the blood is removed and redirected to the bladder to be expelled from the body.

You can confirm this yourself: drink about six glasses of a beverage in one day instead of water. You will notice that your trips to the washroom are more often than regular as you will eliminate at least sixty percent of the liquid you've ingested. In practical terms, this means that if you are going to hydrate your body with other beverages like fruit and vegetable juices. You may need to drink twice as much to get the same results as you would when drinking pure water.

When we drink water along with food, the water mixes with the food and loses its hydrating quality. Pure water should always be taken at least three hours after a meal, when there is no more food in the stomach, or one hour before eating anything, to allow the water to clear the stomach.

If we try to hydrate our cells by drinking lots of juices, teas, coffee, or sodas, the process will not be very effective. I'm not saying that these juices are not good for drinking, as they may be great as food or medicine, but not for *hydrating* the cells of the body.

Some drinks such as coffee, black tea, cocoa, and colas have toxins like caffeine in them that must be diluted with large quantities of water to be flushed from the body. These drinks have the potential to contribute large amounts of water, but a big portion of this water must be used to eliminate the toxins they contain. The only contribution they bring to the body is intoxication.

Artificial sweeteners in drinks also add to the body's toxic burden. Sugars and caffeine create an acidic environment in the body, impeding proper enzyme function and overloading the kidneys, which must rid the body of this excess acid (Experience Life 2010). So, as far as hydration is concerned, it is best to rely on pure water.

What about drinking warm water in the morning? It is advised that water be taken at body temperature. However, if you live in an environment where temperatures are generally cooler, room temperature is usually below body temperature and in such cases, it would be smart to warm the water a little. Furthermore, drinking warm water is also beneficial to health, especially for those suffering from Hashimoto. It helps to warm the body of those who have hypothyroidism, whose bodies are usually cold.

Many people recommend squeezing lemon juice into a glass of warm water in the morning. Lemon juice is very beneficial, but the lemon converts the pure water into a food element, eliminating its hydrating property, so it all depends on what we hope to receive from the things we ingest.

To receive the best benefits, drink water the way nature designed it: unaltered (no chlorine, fluoride or any other additive).

Carbohydrates

Carbohydrates are the sugars, starches, and fibers found in fruits, grains, vegetables and milk products. When you eat carbohydrates, regardless of the source (bread, pasta, rice, cookies, candy, soda and even vegetables and fruits), it turns into glucose the moment it hits your bloodstream.

Recently, there has been a lot of attention given to sugar. It has been dismissed as if there is nothing good about it. However, sugar is not all that bad. It is not only good but essential for the proper functioning of the thyroid gland and the immune system.

I used to believe that sugar was sugar until I was diagnosed with Hashimoto. This then led me to study in more detail the effects of sugar in the body. All sugars are not the same and the body does not metabolize them in the same way. Each sugar has a separate function in the human body, and all sugars are essential for optimum health.

Consider with me the two of the eight essential sugars: glucose and fructose.

Glucose is the energy sugar. It is the fuel that keeps our body working, and all cells of the body need glucose for energy. The problem with glucose is that we consume more than twice the amount needed. The excess sugar is then converted to a cholesterol-producing fat. So, the issue should not be about the evil of glucose but, the evil of our over indulgence.

According to the American Heart Association, the maximum amount of added sugars you should eat in a day is:

- Men: 150 calories per day (37.5 grams or nine teaspoons)

- Women: 100 calories per day (25 grams or six teaspoons)

To put that into perspective, one 12-ounce can of Coke contains 140 calories from sugar, while a regular-sized Snickers bar contains 120 calories from sugar (Gunnars 2016).

Regular sugar or table sugar is a disaccharide made up of fifty percent glucose and fifty percent fructose (Encyclopedia Britannica: Sucrose). Most of us can easily meet the daily recommended allowance by eliminating refined sugar from our diets, including all sweetened processed drinks.

Fructose, in contrast to glucose, is not used in the body to produce energy. It is beneficial to the body for blood sugar control, for fetal health, and for the control of body weight, blood pressure, uric acid, and cholesterol. It should be taken in moderate amounts, especially by those who suffer from Hashimoto thyroiditis.

Excess fructose is metabolized in the liver and converted into VLDL, the damaging form of cholesterol and fatty acids. Fructose increases the body's ability to store fat, most of which is stored in the liver. Metabolizing fructose overloads the liver and causes liver damage like that caused by too much alcohol.

During the metabolism of fructose, uric acid is produced, which in high amounts, could lead to high blood pressure, kidney stones, and gout. Fructose promotes the growth of bad bacteria, interferes with the development and growth in infants and children, and impairs long-term memory. Too much fructose also causes the mineralization of teeth, leading to tooth decay. It is the main food for cancer cells, accelerating their growth and spreading ability. Fructose also quickens the aging process and damages the lining of the small intestines, which leads to digestion and absorption problems.

So, is fructose a bad sugar to be avoided at all cost? No, but special control needs to be exercised when consuming it. It is worth recalling, too, that an excess of fructose produces insulin resistance. When this happens, the energy level in the body falls. The pituitary gland, becoming aware that the body is low in energy, interprets this data as if the body is low on insulin, so it releases cortisol to prompt the pancreas to make more insulin, flooding the body with more cortisol. This abundance of cortisol and insulin is detrimental to the thyroid gland, causing it to become more inflamed. Thus, controlling the ingestion of fructose is a key factor in healing the immune system and reviving a supposedly "dead" thyroid gland.

Even health-conscious individuals could overdose on fructose if he or she consistently eats a lot of fruits. Too much of a good thing could be bad for you.

While many of the studies into this subject are obscure, a growing body of research suggests that greater than fifty grams of fructose a day is detrimental. Some suggest that twenty-five grams should be the limit, and for people with known metabolic syndrome or its risk factors, fifteen grams is the limit (Tieman 2016; Johnson and Murray 2010).

Regular table sugar is fifty percent glucose and fifty percent fructose. Most processed foods contain a high content of fructose— approximately fifty-five percent fructose and forty-five percent glucose. Fructose is also abundant in fruits and some vegetables; hence there is no difficulty for us to over-consume this sugar. The key thing to realize is that while every cell in the body can use glucose, the liver is the only organ that can metabolize fructose in significant amounts.

Fructose not only leads to gradual weight increase, it also boosts the activity of the stress hormone, cortisol. Serbian biochemists have demonstrated this effect in rats that were given fructose water to drink (Biljana et al. 2013).

At first glance, cortisol and insulin appear to have opposite effects. Insulin is a storage hormone. Under high insulin levels, the body stores energy in the form of glycogen and fat. Cortisol, on the other hand, prepares the body for action. This moves energy out of stores and into readily available forms, such as glucose.

Excess fructose stimulates the production of cortisol which produces glucose, normally to be used for vigorous physical exertion. When this does not happen, *glucose levels remain high*. This chronic elevation in glucose *trigger the release of insulin*. Chronically elevated cortisol leads to adrenal fatigue. (Tanja et al., 2010).

Dr. Mercola recommends limiting your total carbohydrate intake to 15 grams per day until your immune problem is resolved. The easiest way to accomplish this is by swapping processed foods; all forms of sugar — particularly fructose — as well as grains, for ideally fresh, whole organic foods. This means cooking from scratch with fresh ingredients. (Dr. Mercola).

Fats

Fats are important for our overall heath. While bad fats can increase your risk of certain diseases, good fats are vital to your physical and emotional health.

Dietary fat is of interest to researchers because fatty acids influence glucose metabolism by altering cell membrane function, enzyme activity, insulin signaling, and gene expression. The evidence of many of these studies suggests that replacing saturated fats and trans fatty acids with unsaturated fats have beneficial effects on insulin sensitivity and are likely to reduce the risk of type 2 diabetes (Ulf et al., 2008).

It is recommended to stay away from processed fat sources like canola oil, corn oil, soybean oil, safflower oil, sesame seed oil, cottonseed oil, vegetable oil, shortening, and margarine. Also, any oil that has been hydrogenated or partially hydrogenated; they are trans-fat and should be avoided (Dietitian Cassie).

Among polyunsaturated fats, linoleic acid from the omega-6 series improves insulin sensitivity. On the other hand, long-chain fatty acids do not improve insulin sensitivity or glucose metabolism (Ulf et al., 2008).

The most recent scientific studies suggest that healthy fats (saturated and unsaturated fats from whole food, animal, and plant sources) should comprise anywhere from 50 to 85 percent of your overall energy (calorie) intake (J. Julie et al., 2013).

According to Dietitian Cassie and other health experts, as a person with diabetes, your goal should not be to increase your insulin requirement by consuming carbohydrates but to decrease it by consuming more healthy fats.

It's easy to consume fewer carbohydrates when you pair them with fat; fats fill you up. Thus, generally, when you eat fat, you eat fewer carbohydrates. By consuming fewer carbohydrates, you are giving your pancreas a break, allowing your body to heal because you require less insulin.

People with diabetes can also benefit more from nutrients like vitamins A, D, E and K for blood sugar support; they all need fat for their absorption into the body.

For diabetics, a good starting point is having two to three tablespoons of fat, every single time you eat—meals and snacks!

The best fats to consume are butter, olive oil, nuts, seeds, cheese, heavy cream, nut butter, avocados, coconut, coconut oil, coconut cream and fat from organic, grass-fed meat. Eat as much high-quality healthy fat as you want.

Remember, fat is high in calories (9 calories per gram) while being small in terms of volume. So, when you look at your plate, the largest portion would be vegetables, not fats (Dr. Mercola).

Improve your omega-3 to omega-6 ratio. Today's Western diet has far too many processed, damaged omega-6 fats, and too little omega-3 fats. The main sources of omega-6 fats are corn, soy, canola, safflower, peanut, and sunflower oil.

The optimal ratio of omega-6 to omega-3 is 1:1. However, our ratio has deteriorated to between 20:1 and 50:1 in favor of omega-6. This lopsided ratio has seriously adverse health consequences (Dr. Mercola).

To remedy this, reduce your consumption of vegetable oils (this means not cooking with them and avoiding processed foods), and increase your intake of animal-based omega-3, such as krill or salmon oil. Vegetable-based omega-3 is also found in flaxseed oil and walnut oil, and it's good to include these in your diet as well. Keep in mind that vegetable omega-3 cannot take the place of *animal-based* omega-3s; they are different.

Coconut: The benefits of coconut for thyroid problems come from its unique medium-chain fatty acids, also known as medium-chain triglycerides or fatty acids. They are characterized by a specific chemical structure that allows the body to absorb them whole. This makes them more easily digestible. Your body processes them as it would carbohydrates, and they are used as a source of direct energy. Medium chain fatty acids are known to increase metabolism and promote weight loss. Coconut oil can also raise basal body temperatures while increasing metabolism (David Wolfe, Eat one tablespoon coconut oil 2016) (The journal of nutrition 2002).

- Lauric acid has excellent anti-inflammatory and antimicrobial properties. It comprises about half of the fatty acid content in coconut milk and oil. Lauric acid is used for treating viral infections including influenza, swine flu, avian flu, the common cold, fever blisters, cold sores, genital herpes caused by herpes simplex virus, genital warts caused by human papillomavirus, and HIV/AIDS. It is also used for preventing the transmission of HIV from mothers to children.

  Other uses for lauric acid include treatment of bronchitis, gonorrhea, yeast infections, chlamydia, intestinal infections caused by a parasite called Giardia lamblia, and ringworm (WebMD lauric acid 2016).

- Capric acids have potent antimicrobial and antiviral properties. It comprises 10% of coconut oil. Capric acid is converted into monocaprin in the body, where it can help combat viruses, bacteria, and the yeast Candida albicans (Livestrong- benefits of capric acid 2015).

- Caprylic acid boasts a good deal of health benefits thanks to its anti-fungal and antibacterial properties. It is used to treat yeast infections, skin conditions, digestive disorders, and high cholesterol (Healthline. Caprylic acid 2016).

The fresh coconut is the best source, but if it is not possible to obtain, virgin coconut oil is the second choice.

Superfood for the thyroid

Bee pollen has been touted as a complete food, containing all the essential nutrients to sustain life, perfect for reversing poor nutrition (Mercola. Bee pollen as Super-food 2016). It is richer in protein than any animal source and is loaded with calcium, phosphorus, magnesium, sodium, potassium, iron, copper, zinc, manganese, silicon, selenium, vitamins (A, E, D, C, and B complex), and folic acid. It is also rich in fatty acids, enzymes, carotenoids, and bioflavonoids (Bee Pollen Buzz 2016).

Bee pollen reduces the presence of histamine by inhibiting the activation of mast cells, making it one of nature's best anti-allergy compounds. It also boasts of extending longevity and boosting the immune system, as well as being antibacterial, antimicrobial, antiviral, antifungal, and an antioxidant. One or two teaspoons daily is all you need to enjoy its health benefits (Mercola 2016).

Moringa oleifera is a plant that has been praised for thousands of years for its health benefits. It has eighteen amino acids, including the nine essential ones. Its anti-inflammatory and antioxidant bioactive compounds are isothiocyanates, flavonoids, phenolic acid, vitamins C and E, beta-carotene, quercetin, and chlorogenic acid (Arnarson 2016).

Zeatin, quercetin, beta-sitosterol, caffeoylquinic acid, and kaempferol are some of its phytonutrients that make Moringa antitumor, antiepileptic, antiulcer, antispasmodic, antihypertensive, and antidiabetic. It is also high in anti-aging, immune-boosting, and thyroid-healing compounds.

Moringa has the distinction of slowing the conversion of T4 to T3, so most health care providers consider it to be ideal for treating Graves' disease, but not good for Hashimoto sufferers. The slightly slower conversion rate of T4 into T3 happens in the individual cells of the body, not in the thyroid gland. This means that whether the thyroid gland is hypothyroid or hyperthyroid, it remains unaffected by this transition (Kar and Tahiliani 2000). The takeaway point is that Moringa benefits the gland by helping to balance its operation and does not adversely affect the gland itself in any way. Two teaspoons of the powdered leaf daily are enough (Arnarson 2016).

Goji is a berry grown in the Himalayan, and in the wild, pristine lowland fertile soil of the Ningxia Province of China. Goji has the highest concentration of antioxidants in the plant kingdom. One of the world's most powerful anti-aging food source, it has a complete spectrum of antioxidants, zeaxanthin, and carotenoids. It is loaded with omega-6, an excellent hormone regulator. It also boasts all the essential amino acids and twenty-one trace minerals, containing a good supply of iron, calcium, zinc, selenium, germanium, phosphorus, vitamins (C, B_1, B_2, B_6), and carotenoids, making Goji antioxidant, antibacterial, anti-inflammatory, and immune system boosting.

A quarter cup of Goji daily is a healthy amount to work with (Patel 2014).

Quinoa, the sacred food of the Incas, could be eaten in place of rice. It packs all nine essential amino acids, along with calcium, phosphorus, sodium, copper, iron, manganese, zinc, and magnesium. The flavonoids quercetin and kaempferol are just two of its antioxidant compounds, while polysaccharides like arabinans, hydroxycinnamic acids, hydroxybenzoic acids, and oleanic acids are a few of its anti-inflammatory phytonutrients.

Quinoa should be on the list of any healthy antioxidant and anti-inflammatory diet (Ware 2016).

Chia seed, a South American giant among food, packs a powerful nutritional punch. It is rich in fiber and has twenty amino acids, including all the essential ones. There is no shortage of calcium, manganese, phosphorus, magnesium, sulfur, iron, niacin, and vitamins A, B, E, and D in it.

Quercetin, kaempferol, chlorogenic acid, and caffeic acid are four of its powerful antioxidants. A chia seed tends to swell once it encounters water, so you don't need a lot. One to two tablespoons a day is enough (Dr. Axe 2016).

Hemp seed is the most nutritious seed and a perfect food (Pure Healing Foods 2016). It promotes cardiovascular health and balances hormones with its content of omega-3 and omega-6 fatty acids. Hemp is also beneficial in alleviating skin allergies. It contains twenty amino acids, including the essential ones, and is loaded with antioxidants, essential fats, and enzymes necessary to promote rapid recovery from disease. Not to mention the gamma-linolenic acids, phospholipids, and phytosterols, the phytonutrients that make this seed an ideal anti-inflammatory super-food.

Four tablespoons daily are the recommended allowance.

Wheatgrass juice contains ninety-eight nutrients, the full vitamin B complex spectrum, all the essential amino acids, vitamins, minerals, enzymes, phytonutrients, and antioxidants. Combined, they protect the body from radiation and inflammation, build the immune system, and stimulate the thyroid gland.

Two ounces of fresh wheatgrass juice a day is ideal (The Chalkboard 2013).

Flax seed made my list of anti-inflammatory Super-foods because it is a rich source of the omega-3 fatty acid, a powerful anti-inflammatory agent. Among plants, it is one of the highest sources of polyphenol and lignan, excellent for balancing hormones. This seed is also anti-aging and good for eliminating bad bacteria.

Flax holds its own as a potent antioxidant. It is also a good source of fiber, protein, vitamins B_1 and B_6, magnesium, manganese, phosphorus, selenium, iron, potassium, copper, and zinc.

These benefits could be enjoyed with three tablespoons of grounded flax seed daily (The World's Healthiest Foods 2016).

Organic apple cider vinegar is the fermented juice of apples. It contains pectin, vitamins (A, B_6, C, E), thiamine, riboflavin, niacin, pentatonic acid, beta-carotene, lycopene, and minerals (such as sodium, phosphorus, potassium, calcium, iron, and magnesium). Add to this list acetic acid, lactic acid, citric acid, and malic acid.

Apple cider vinegar made this list because of its anti-inflammatory and anti-allergy properties (Underground health reporter 2016).

Some preliminary research suggests that apple cider vinegar may benefit people with type 2 diabetes, high blood pressure, and weight loss problems (Buller, Johnston, and Kim 2004). It may also help to prevent the overgrowth of *Malassezia furfur,* the bacteria that trigger dandruff. Apple cider vinegar is also credited with helping to alleviate allergies though no scientific evidence proves that claim (Grumman Bender 2014).

Apple cider vinegar made this list because of its anti-inflammatory and anti-allergy properties (Underground health reporter 2016).

A word of caution: vinegar could eat away at the enamel on teeth, so it should be well-diluted. Do not use it as a mouth rinse. One tablespoon mixed into eight ounces of juice or water is suggested (Mercola 2015).

The illnesses that are treated with these Super-foods, run into the hundreds. In this list, I limited myself to mentioning only the properties from which Hashimoto sufferers will benefit most. The nutrients in these foods were designed to correct any malfunction of the immune system, thyroid, the adrenal gland, and the entire body once they are integrated into the lifestyle.

These plants were placed on this earth with the sole purpose of nurturing the body and healing not only the ills we know and feel, but also those that we just can't put a finger on.

Super-foods are loaded with nutrients in the proper ratios ready to be utilized by organs and systems of the body to promote good health. It is virtually impossible to overcome Hashimoto thyroiditis without the help of these super-foods. They provide us with all the nutrients that the body needs to maintain itself as disease-free.

In short, we have in these simple foods all the raw material to fight off any illness and live without the disease. These super-foods are nutritious, anti-inflammatory, antioxidant, antifungal, antibacterial, antiviral, and immune-boosting and regulating—the perfect recipe for healing!

Minerals

Minerals are an essential part of the human body. Minerals are just as vital as vitamins in keeping your body healthy. In fact, mineral deficiencies can lead to a host of health problems.

Ensuring your diet is rich in the following minerals, will help you restore balance and reduce the need for thyroid medications.

Zinc: research indicates that zinc is something that people with diabetes should think about. The body can't make zinc, so we must take it in from food sources. Zinc is stored in the muscles, blood cells, the retina of the eye, skin, bone, kidney, liver, pancreas, and in men, prostate.

Symptoms of zinc deficiency include stunted growth (in children), hair loss, diarrhea, decreased appetite, eye, and skin lesions, delayed wound healing, and weight loss. People with chronic gastrointestinal disorders, such as Crohn disease, are at risk for zinc deficiency (Amy Campbell, MS, RD, LDN, CDE. 2007).

If you have a zinc deficiency, then animal foods are better sources of zinc than plant foods. The best *sources* of *zinc* are seafood, meat, seeds, and cooked dried beans, peas and lentils.

The daily recommended dose of zinc is 12 mg for women and 15 mg for men. Zinc lozenges, particularly in the form of zinc gluconate, are a good source of zinc because they are readily absorbable (Beletate et al., 2007).

Iron is required for thyroid hormone production, the conversion of T4 into T3 and for the best utilization of T3 inside the cell.

Iodine is required for thyroid hormone production in the gland. Eating foods rich in iodine, such as seaweed and seafood, can provide enough iodine. The recommended minimum iodine intake for most adults is 150 micrograms a day, according to the Office of Dietary Supplements. Good food sources include milk, cheese, poultry, eggs, kelp, and other seaweeds.

Selenium This is a crucial component of the enzyme that converts T4 to T3 in the body. Without it, T3 cannot be produced in the right amounts, and organs will function as if they were hypothyroid even though blood test levels are normal. Foods that provide selenium include tuna, shrimp, salmon, sardines, scallops, lamb, chicken, beef, turkey, eggs, and shitake mushrooms. Or you can take 100 to 200 micrograms of selenium in supplement form per day.

T4 is the inactive thyroid hormone; it must be converted into T3, which is the active form of thyroid hormone before it can be used by the body. On the surface of each cell there is a nuclear receptor where thyroid hormone T3 binds, and then we have energy.

To manufacture T4 the body needs iodine, vitamin B2, Vitamin C. Your best sources of iodine are fresh vegetables, seafood, kelp, and seaweed.

For converting the inactive T4 into the active form T3, the body needs Selenium, vitamin D, and Vitamin A. These ten nutrients are required in the process of getting your body energized. Any deficiency of these nutrients and the improvement of the thyroid will be minimal (Peter Osborne).

Vitamins

Vitamins help to regulate chemical reactions in the body. There are 13 vitamins, including vitamins A, B complex, C, D, E, and K. Most vitamins cannot be made in the body, so we must obtain them through the diet. Vitamins are best consumed through a varied diet rather than as a supplement because it reduces the chances of taking too high a dose.

Vitamin A: Many Hashimoto's patients are deficient in Vitamin A. This will limit the body to convert thyroid T4 hormone into its usable T3 form and could lead to on-going hypothyroidism; even if you are on medication.

Vitamin A also activates the gene that regulates Thyroid Stimulating Hormone (TSH)

A study published in 2012 by the *Journal of the American College of Nutrition* looked at how 25,000 IU a day of Vitamin A supplementation improved the conversion rate of T4 to T3 in pre-menopausal women. At the end of the 4 months trial these were the results (Farhangi et al.):

- 30% to 33% reduction in TSH.
- 38% to 61% increase in T3 thyroid hormone.
- 16% to 23% decrease in T4 thyroid hormone.

The vitamin A used in this research study was different from the vitamin A that you are familiar with.

We associate Vitamin A, with carrots, a rich source of beta-carotene; which is a form of Vitamin A. The liver must convert beta-carotene into Vitamin A before your body can use it. However, this conversion is not very efficient among those suffering from Hashimoto. So even though you may be eating lots of beta-carotene in your diet, you could still be Vitamin A deficient.

If your body is unable to do this conversion effectively as is the case with Hashimoto, you'll either need to include animal foods in your meal plan or obtain retinoid forms of vitamin A through dietary supplements.

B vitamins are a class of water-soluble chemicals that cells need to carry on normal physiological functions. A deficiency in B-vitamins, more specifically B2, B3, B6, B12 and B9 (folate) can lead to hypothyroidism. Folate is also important as it ties in closely with TSH levels.

Vitamins B6 and B12 support nerve health, which is critical for addressing conditions such as diabetic neuropathy. Biotin is another B-complex vitamin that is necessary for both metabolism and growth. Biotin is also involved in the manufacture and utilization of protein, fats, and carbohydrates (Dr. Julian Whitaker).

Thiamine B1 is a water-soluble vitamin that functions to convert blood sugar into energy. It helps with digestion, cardiovascular and muscular function, as well as keeping mucous membranes healthy. Thiamine is found in various food sources such as pork, eggs, legumes, peas, nuts, and whole-grain cereals. Thiamine deficiency causes many symptoms such as depression, irritability, abdominal pain, weakness, and fatigue.

Researchers have suggested that people with autoimmune diseases may have an enzymatic imbalance which affects the body's ability to process thiamine. The recommended dose is about 1.1 milligrams/day for women and 1.5 milligrams/day for men (Naomi Parker)

B2 (Riboflavin) Deficiency of Vitamin B2 suppresses thyroid function in that the thyroid and adrenal glands fail to secrete their hormones.

The current DV for Riboflavin (Vitamin B2) is 1.7mg. Sources of vitamin B2 are milk, crimini mushrooms, leafy green vegetables, turkey, sardines, and eggs, Legumes, peppers, root vegetables, and squash,

Niacinamide (vitamin B_3), also known as nicotinamide, is one of two principal forms of the B-complex vitamin. Vitamin B_3 is found in many foods including yeast, meat, fish, milk, eggs, green vegetables, beans, and cereal grains. Niacin and niacinamide are also found in many vitamin B complex supplements. Niacinamide can be made from niacin in the body. Niacin is converted to niacinamide when it is taken in amounts greater than what is needed by the body (Dietitians of Canada).

Niacinamide naturally improves endothelial cell function, which is one of the key pieces of the puzzle in cell regeneration. Niacinamide is required for the proper metabolizing of fats and sugars in the body and to maintain healthy cells (Hubert Kolb et al.).

The recommended daily allowance for niacin is 16 mg/day for men and 14 mg/day for women. Some of the sources rich in niacinamide are Brewer's yeast, beef liver, chicken, pork, salmon, tuna, swordfish, and turkey. Peanuts, sunflower seeds, and halibut are other useful foods to avail this nutrient. Beets and green vegetables contain vitamin B3. The vitamin is also found in legumes, such as lentils, lima beans, and peanuts.

The US Recommended Dietary Allowances for Niacinamide is 20 mg per day in general to benefit the diabetic (Diabetes information; Dr. Axe B3).

Vitamin B6, also called pyridoxine, is a water-soluble nutrient that is part of the B-vitamin family. B6 helps support adrenal function, calm and maintain a healthy nervous system and are necessary for key metabolic processes. Vitamin B6 acts as a coenzyme in the breakdown and utilization of carbohydrates, fats, and proteins.

The best sources of vitamin B_6 include meat, fish, poultry, organ meats, enriched cereals and meatless soy products, nuts, lentils and some vegetables and fruit (Larry Armstrong).

According to the National Institutes of Health, the U.S. Recommended Daily Allowance for adult males between

19 and 50 years of age is 1.3 mg, and those over the age of 50 need 1.7 mg. Women between 19 and 50 years of age should take 1.3 mg, and those over 50 should take 1.5 mg. Pregnant women should take 1.9 mg and lactating women, 2 mg.

Dr. Weil recommends 50 mg as part of a daily B-complex supplement that contains a full spectrum of B vitamins, including thiamin, B12, riboflavin, and niacin.

Vitamin C, also known as L-ascorbic acid, is a water-soluble vitamin that is naturally present in some foods, added to others, and available as a supplement. Humans, unlike most animals, are unable to synthesize vitamin C, so it is an essential dietary component (Li Y, Schellhorn HE 2007).

It is common to find those with thyroid disease to be low or deficient in Vitamin C. Vitamin C supports the immune system and is needed to produce thyroid hormone, increase fruit and vegetable intake to increase the amount of this for better metabolic activity.

High vitamin C foods include bell peppers, dark leafy greens, kiwifruit, broccoli, berries, citrus fruits, tomatoes, peas, and papayas.

Vitamin D is a fat-soluble *vitamin* that is naturally present in very few foods. *Vitamin D* promotes calcium absorption in the gut, helps to modulate the immune system and has been shown to be useful for preventing autoimmune thyroid diseases. To do this, vitamin D binds to specific receptors on certain immune cells and prevent them from destroying the cells of the thyroid gland. The kinds of immune cells affected by vitamin D include monocytes, natural killer cells as well as T and B cells.

Vitamin D is oil soluble, which means you need to eat fat to absorb it. Foods high in vitamin D include fish, mushrooms, tofu, yogurt, milk, milk substitutes, fortified breakfast cereals, orange juice, pork chops, and eggs.

Vitamin D is also naturally made by the body when the skin is exposed to the sun. Depending on where you live, 20 minutes of sun exposure a day is enough to meet your vitamin D requirement.

Tocotrienols are members of the vitamin *E* family. Vitamin E is composed of eight different compounds. Half of these are called *tocopherols*, which is the most common form of vitamin E. The other half are known as *tocotrienols.* While both tocopherols and tocotrienols do occur in nature, there is no plant that provides the entire family of tocopherols and tocotrienols in adequate amounts.

Tocotrienols are potent antioxidants, which appear to reduce the oxidant-induced inflammation that contributes to bone loss. Tocotrienols also up-regulate genes related to new bone formation while suppressing inflammatory signaling that generates bone destruction. There is also compelling evidence of Tocotrienol effectiveness in treating non-alcoholic fatty liver disease (Thomas Rosenthal 2014).

Rice bran oil, wheat germ, barley, oats, coconut oil and palm kernel oil all contain one or more types of tocotrienols as well, however, only palm fruit oil contain all four types. Palm fruit oil is composed of 30 percent tocopherols and 70 percent tocotrienols. The oil is extracted from the fleshy mesocarp of the palm fruit and is useful in a myriad of food preparations. It is said to be the most widely used oil in the world, perhaps because it is more heat stable than other vegetable oils and provides superior taste and texture qualities (Jiyeon Chuna, et al.).

The Food and Nutrition Board of the Institute of Medicine in the United States and the National Academy of Sciences have no definition for the health benefits or risks, including Estimated Average Requirement, Recommended Dietary Allowance, Adequate Intake, or Tolerable Upper Intake Level, associated with tocotrienols.

Standard dosages can fall between 140 to 360 mg/day, but the more common dosages fall within the 40 to 50 mg/day range. Generally, there are no differences in dosage among children and adults, though children under the age of 10 are advised not to use tocotrienols at all unless under the recommendation of a physician.

Since tocotrienols are derived from vitamin E, there are no known side effects, even when dosages are as high as 2500 mg/day per kilogram in the body.

Spices

Ginger has a very long history of use in various forms of alternative medicine. It has been used to help digestion, reduce nausea and help fight the flu and common cold, to name a few.

The main components are gingerol, beta-carotene, capsaicin, caffeic acid, salicylate, and niacin. Together they suppress the immune system cells that are responsible for the production of pro-inflammatory chemicals. It also promotes sweating, a perfect aid for detoxification.

The *"Journal of Microbiology and Antimicrobials"* published a study in 2011 that tested just how effective ginger is in enhancing immune function against *Staphylococcus aureus* and *Streptococcus pyrogens* as opposed to conventional antibiotics.

These Nigerian researchers discovered that the natural solution from ginger was more effective than the drugs — chloramphenicol, ampicillin, and tetracycline. This is important because these two bacteria cause complications to already immune-compromised patients (A. Sebiomo et al. 2011).

Ginger's main components are gingerol, beta-carotene, capsaicin, caffeic acid, salicylate, and niacin. Together they suppress the cytokines and chemokines, immune system cells that are responsible for the production of pro-inflammatory chemicals. It also promotes sweating, a perfect aid for detoxification (World's Healthiest Foods 2016).

Cinnamon is a sweet spice. Its main compound, cinnamaldehyde, is responsible for its antifungal, antiviral, and antibacterial properties, but it may also kill good bacteria, so regular replenishment with probiotics is recommended.

Cinnamon extract seems to be very effective in preventing HIV from entering cells. Along with being anticarcinogenic, this spice has a high concentration of antioxidant and anti-inflammatory compounds (Leech 2016).

A word of caution: there are many kinds of cinnamon. The two main varieties are cassia and Ceylon. Cassia is cheaper and more popular, but the health benefits mentioned above are attributed to Ceylon, which is the true cinnamon. One teaspoon maximum daily is recommended for the first four weeks.

Almost Home

Hashimoto Thyroiditis is a multi-factor disease involving different organs and systems in the body. Each one of them must be addressed before we can see any significant improvement of the illness.

There are many theories as to what causes Hashimoto. However, when we consider all the scientific evidence available to us; I believe that we could easily narrow it down to one: *nutritional imbalance.*

Some of us have a monotonous diet; we eat the same foods day in and day out. So, we are receiving the same nutrients consistently every day. We then end up with so much of certain nutrients, that they become toxic to our bodies, while been deficient in others. This means that our initial response to this illness should be to re-establish this delicate balance of nutrients. These nutrients are the building blocks of health; the raw material the body needs to get its built-in self-healing ability in motion.

We may not know exactly what is causing the destruction of the thyroid. But, the one thing we do know is that most offenders enter our body through our digestive system. If we could block the entrance, the disease will cease to exist, even if you do not know what exactly was coming in.

We have an amazing digestive system, which will ensure that only the right chemicals that the body needs, gets into circulation. So, our first step in the battle against Diabetes should be to make sure that this system is working properly.

The scientific community has enlightened us in terms of the many specific nutrients that could be used to treat each of the many factors involved in the progression of Hashimoto Thyroiditis.

We can win against this disease! But we must attack it like an avalanche from all sides with every, Hashimoto's destroying nutrients; then it won't be long before you will find yourself free from its shackles.

Health can only be obtained, by the regular consumption of every known essential nutrient along with their cofactors, whose greatest concentrations exist in nutrient dense super-foods.

You may not know the exact cause of your disease. However, that does not imply that it cannot be treated successfully. If you follow the basic principles of healthy living, you could keep any disease at bay.

Your fight against Hashimoto Thyroiditis should include curcumin as your number one weapon. Curcumin has the distinction of being able to down-regulate the immune system by limiting the expression of the CD24 gene. This gene is responsible for the increase of Macrophage and the antibody-producing B cells. As the number of these cell decreases, so will the autoimmune disease.

Curcumin has the property that it can also contribute to the regeneration of the thyroid gland even after severe mutilation as consequence of Hashimoto Thyroiditis. It is effective as a treatment during every stage of recovery.

Second on the list are the adrenals, the thyroid's best friend. The adrenals secrete cortisol; the fire extinguishers of the body. We know that consistently high level of cortisol could cause hypothyroidism, but low levels of cortisol could cause Hashimoto thyroiditis.

When the adrenals have been producing high amounts of cortisol for a long period, eventually, they burn out and we end up with adrenal insufficiency. This reduced production of cortisol is not enough to control inflammation in the body, so it rages on indefinitely as an autoimmune disease.

These autoimmune diseases will rage on as long as the adrenals are under-performing. For this reason, healing the adrenals must be a top priority. If we win the battle in restoring the adrenals, we win the war against Hashimoto disease.

The number one producer of cortisol and cause of adrenal insufficiency is stress. Stress is difficult to combat because the things that produce stress in our lives are the things we love to hold close: fear, doubt, hate, anger, frustration, jealousy, envy, malice, vengeance, disappointment, and worries of all sorts. Deep down, if we harbor just one of these negative emotions, it is enough to prolong our stress.

Ongoing stress means continued adrenal fatigue and the perpetuation of Hashimoto. So, I hope you see why engaging in some type of relaxation discipline works to our advantage.

Another prime cause of adrenal insufficiency is sugar consumption. Fructose, a constituent of regular sugar, is not used in the body in large quantity. The liver uses fructose, it is bacteria-favored food, and the rest of it stimulates the adrenals to secrete cortisol. Given the large amount of sugar that we consume in our daily diet, it should be easy to see why it could pose a problem for us.

Some tender loving care for the adrenals could go a long way. For us to have adequate cortisol levels and put the fires of inflammation out in our body, the adrenals must have time to rest and recover. So, closely monitor your sugar intake and stress levels; it is crucial!

Next, you will want to focus your attention on lectins. Although the body could handle a fair amount of these offenders; we run into problems because of over-consumption. Consider how much potatoes or wheat you eat daily! In most cases, it is not about the lectin but the amount that we consume. Take a close look at your diet. It may be that you are eating too much milk, tomato, or some other food. Your keywords should be moderation and balance in your diet. Test the food; if it does not make you feel better or if it makes you feel worse, don't eat it. It is your health, so you need to take control.

Lectin, like gliadin, binds itself with trans-glutaminase and irritates the cells of the thyroid gland, inducing an immune response which results in more inflammation. Gliadin may not be the sole cause of damages to the thyroid gland, but it is a strong contributor. Thus, our best course of action is to abstain from eating gluten for the time being.

Do not under-estimate the power of goitrogen. Here, you want to proceed with absolute caution. Remember, you are afflicted with an autoimmune disease, your thyroid gland is mutilated and under-performing to say the least. Every bit of goitrogen you consume will slow it even further.

After Hashimoto goes into remission, a little goitrogen may be helpful to get the thyroid gland to grow or regenerate new cells to the point where it once again gives you enough hormone to get you through the day with enough energy. However, to reap that benefit, at some point, you will have to stop consuming the goitrogen. If a food is not helping you to recover, what is the point of eating it?

Remember, goitrogens are only partially destroyed by cooking, while others like soy goitrogen are enhanced by heat.

Most people have some form of allergy. Get yourself tested; you may have hidden allergies that you know nothing about; they can be making you sick. Histamine is released by the immune system in response to allergens (some of which are airborne pollen, dust mites, mold, animal dander, or certain proteins in food). Even if you tested negative for allergies, be careful, as a negative result does not mean that you don't have any allergies.

You may have mild allergic reactions that do not affect normal individuals, but they could add up to big problems if you are afflicted with Hashimoto.

With an inflamed thyroid gland, every drop of histamine—even if it does not provoke an allergic symptom—contributes to making the inflammation in the gland chronic. It's like alcohol: rub it on your skin and it does nothing, but put a drop of it on an open wound and it burns like hell. That is what histamine does to inflammation.

To effectively manage histamine levels, you will need to keep an eye for all allergens and all histamine-containing and histamine-producing foods and avoid them.

There is no escaping genetically modified food in North America, but we still need to have a plan of action.

The most manipulated and unhealthy foods are those of animal origin. The chemicals added to the foods that are fed to these animals are toxic to the human body. These chemicals are not intended to support good health but are used to increase production.

You also would be better off by eliminating food derived from hybrid plants. These plants were not genetically modified but were genetically manipulated through cross-pollination or grafting. Although chemicals have not been used in the process, human manipulation does alter the delicate balance of nutrients in these foods (as is the case of wheat, rye, barley, and other gluten-containing foods).

Consider a horse and a donkey. Crossbreed them and we end up with a mule, an animal that is good for work, but useless for procreation. The same thing happens with plants—they lose their life-giving properties through genetic manipulation.

Unfortunately, almost every plant-based product found in North American supermarkets has been, to some extent, modified or manipulated genetically with the sole purpose of appealing to your appetite. So, all the self-conscious efforts on your part to eat healthy have already been sabotaged. For this reason, we cannot rely on supermarket-bought products in our endeavor to recover from any chronic disease. We need to find a better source for the healing nutrients that we need

We need to consider a change in the choice of the food we consume. We need to educate our taste buds to savor and appreciate food that will bring well-being, which promotes life and overall health. Thus, we must resort to a plant-based diet of super foods, most of which could be found on the shelves of health food stores and have not undergone the process of genetic modification.

There are many differing opinions about diets, it's wise to not get all tangled up as to which one is "best". With Hashimoto, our diet cannot be ready-made, but custom-made. This is not the time to be focusing on vegetarianism, Veganism, or any of the other various -isms. To overcome this disease, you need to concentrate on a balance of foods that will give you the nutrients you need and aid you on your way to recovery.

Maintaining a variety in the food we consume should be one of our main concerns.

The best approach is a diet that consists of seventy-five percent raw foods (like fruits, vegetables, seeds, and nuts) and twenty-five percent cooked food. You may even want to leave some room to eat a piece of fish or maybe chicken. The only extreme measure that one should adopt is abstinence from anything processed, as in any food that comes in cans, boxes, or bags. There is nothing healthy about those kinds of foods. They are nutrient-deficient and histamine-producing.

What else could I say? The process of getting healthy again involves a complete change in lifestyle, which will include getting the proper amount of sleep, water, and exercise; the virtual elimination of all processed food along with some balanced, plant-based diet, rich with super-foods.

A balanced diet with Hashimoto thyroiditis could be very challenging because after limiting lectin and allergen-containing/histamine-producing foods, reducing fructose consumption, and avoiding junk food, goitrogenic substances, and genetically modified food; what's left to eat? A very limited list. And there just aren't enough nutrients in them to maintain a healthy body. This forces us to rely on nutrient-dense food like Hemp, Sesame seed, Goji, and others that I have mentioned in this book. They help to manage inflammation, balance the immune system, rebuild the thyroid and adrenal glands, and remove antibodies.

Be prepared to question your health care provider about this disease, for that kind of relationship is beneficial for recovery.

Once we take control in managing this disease, it will take about six months for the adrenals to recover and the cells of the thyroid to heal. However, even though the inflammation is gone, and the production of antibodies ended, we will still have a hypothyroid condition to deal with. There are three reasons for this:

- The cells of the thyroid have been damaged and need to be regenerated.

- The thyroid gland is covered under a blanket of TSH-blocking antibodies; they need to be removed.

- The adrenals are exhausted and need to be rejuvenated.

One of the big secrets in the medical world, is that the thyroid gland, even if damaged, could regenerate new cells. However, it cannot resume normal production of the thyroid hormone until it is once more being stimulated by thyroid-stimulating hormones. That won't happen until the thyroid-stimulating blocking autoantibodies are cleared from the thyroid gland.

There is no known way to kill these antibodies. Our only alternative is to wait it out. But they do not live forever so that is good news! It will take somewhere between six to eighteen months from the time that the inflammation ceases for these antibodies to die off and leave the way clear for the thyroid-stimulating hormone to resume its job. The thyroid will then spring back to life, and by this time, the adrenal glands will have also recovered and be ready to work.

May I add here that for the thyroid gland to regenerate new cells, it must be stimulated by the TSH hormone or antibodies. If you are taking any form of hormone replacement and you are taking a full dose, this could prevent or slow thyroid regeneration, because Synthroid or armour thyroid will neutralize the thyroid gland, by preventing the production of TSH hormone.

The ideal approach here would be not to take the thyroid supplement, but if you feel inclined to take it, then only take a partial dose. Leave room for the thyroid gland to make up the difference. This will get the body producing the TSH hormone and the thyroid will begin to work again.

You may want to consider taking Resveratrol; it has the property of stimulating the pituitary gland to secrete TSH. And do not be afraid of having a TSH reading a little above normal if you had Hashimoto. It will remain high if the thyroid is not producing thyroid hormone in adequate amount.

The extra TSH will cause the thyroid to enlarge and when the thyroid gland has grown to the point where it can produce its normal share of thyroid hormone the TSH levels will normalize. However. Before that happens, you will need some way to stimulate the pituitary gland to secrete TSH; resveratrol and exercise does that job very well.

During this recovery stage, you will also need Ashwagandha; it helps to restore the adrenals and stimulate the thyroid into production of thyroid hormone.

Do not forget the power of vitamin A. Without it, the body cannot convert T4 into T3. Vitamin A is crucial for this conversion process to take place

You will not make it without some form of moderate exercise. Exercise benefits all the organs and systems of the body and is especially beneficial when trying to revitalize a mutilated thyroid gland.

Patience is required here. Improvement will be slow and gradual, but, it will be steady. There may be weeks, or even months, depending on how loyal you are following in your treatment, when it may seem like the improvements have reached a plateau. You may feel like you aren't getting worse or better, but don't give up. Be vigilant and stick to the plan.

The information I have shared with you in this book, have helped me to by-pass taking the medication, send Hashimoto thyroiditis into remission, and nourish the thyroid gland back to health. I hope you have found it useful!

Thank you for reading!

BIBLIOGRAPHY

1/2CP@cohr. 2015. "Life Is 10% What Happens to Us and 90% How We React to It. - Charles Swindoll," February 27. http://cetrola.global2.vic.edu.au/2015/02/27/life-is-10-what-happens-to-us-and-90-how-we-react-to-it-charles-swindoll/.

A.Sebiomo, A. D. Awofodu, A. O. Awosanya, F. E. Awotona and A. J. Ajayi Comparative studies of antibacterial effect of some antibiotics and ginger (Zingiber officinale) on two pathogenic bacteria. Journal of Microbiology and Antimicrobials Vol. 3(1), pp. 18-22, January 2011 accessed Nov. 08, 2017

Aaltonen, Johanna, Petra Björses, Nina Horelli-Kuitunen, Marie-Laure Yaspo, and Leena Peltonen. 1998. "Gene Defect Behind APECED: A New Clue to Autoimmunity," *Human Molecular Genetics* 7(10) 1547-1553. doi: 10.1093/hmg/7.10.1547.

Abbas, Abul K. and Vinay Kumar. 1999. *Robbins Pathologic Basis of Disease*, 6th ed. Philadelphia: Saunders.

AdrenalFatigue.org. 2016. "Cortisol & Adrenal Function." Accessed October 7. https://adrenalfatigue.org/cortisol-adrenal-function/.

Adrian ASĂNICĂ , Carmen MANOLE, Valerica TUDOR , Andreea DOBRE , Răzvan Ionu□ TEODORESCU, Lycium barbarum L. JUICE - NATURAL SOURCE OF BIOLOGICALLY ACTIVE COMPOUNDS. Agro life journal web. Nov. 08, 2017 Agapov, M.M., L.P. Churilov, A.B. Poletaev, and Y. Stroev. 2012. "Immunophysiology Versus Immunopathology: Natural Autoimmunity in Human Health and Disease," *Pathophysiology*. doi: 10.1016/j.pathophys.2012.07.003.

Akedo, Ikuko, Sanae Fukuda, Itaru Kaji, Kanehisa Morimoto, Tatsuya Ioka, Ryu Ishihara, Hideki Ishikawa, Hiroyuki Narahara, and Noriya Uedo. 2004. "Reduction in Salivary Cortisol Level by Music Therapy during Colonoscopic Examination," *Hepatogastroenterology* 51(56) 451-3. https://www.ncbi.nlm.nih.gov/pubmed/15086180.

Akuzawa, Masako, Masatomo Mori, Masami Murakami, Tetsurou Satoh, Hiroyuki Shimizu, and Masanobu Yamada. 1998. "Preserved Activation of Thyrotropin Receptor Antibody to Stimulate Thyroid Function Despite Long-Term Treatment in Euthyroid Patients With Graves' Disease," *European Journal of Endocrinology* (1998) 138 281-285. http://www.eje-online.org/content/ 138/3/281.full.pdf.

Alegret, Marta, Mireia Farré, Juan Carlos Laguna, Núria Roglans, Rosa María Sánchez, Manuel Vázquez-Carrera, and Laia Vilà. 2007. "Impairment of Hepatic Stat-3 Activation and Reduction of Pparα Activity in Fructose-Fed Rats," *Hepatology* 45(3) 778–788. doi: 10.1002/hep.21499.

Allen LV Jr. 2013 Jan-Feb;17(1):39-44 "Adrenal fatigue."web. Oct. 21, 2017

Alessio Fasano "Zonulin and Its Regulation of Intestinal Barrier Function: The Biological Door to Inflammation, Autoimmunity, and Cancer" http://physrev.physiology.org/content/91/1/151.long

Allison A.C., J. Ferluga, H. Prydz, and H.U. Schorlemmer. 1978. "The Role of Macrophage Activation in Chronic Inflammation," *Agents and Actions* 8(1-2):27-35.https://www.ncbi.nlm.nih.gov/pubmed/345781.

Allison A Brown and, Frank B Hu 2001 "Dietary modulation of endothelial function: implications for cardiovascular disease." Am J Clin Nutr **April 2001** vol. 73 no. 4 **673-686** web. November 08, 2017

Alm, P.E. 1983. "Sodium Fluoride Evoked Histamine Release From Mast Cells. A Study of Cyclic AMP Levels and Effects of Catecholamines," *Agents and Actions* 13(2-3):132-7. https://www.ncbi.nlm.nih.gov/pubmed/6191542.

Alterio, Daniela, Bianca Gibelli, Barbara A. Jereczek-Fossa, Jacek Jassem, Roberto Orecchia, and Nicoletta Tradati. 2004. "Radiotherapy-Induced Thyroid Disorders," *Cancer Treatment Reviews* 30(4) 369-384. doi: 10.1016/j.ctrv.2003.12.003.John Lazarus, MA, MD, FRCP, FRCOG, FACE; Dr James Hennessey, M.D., *https://web.archive.org/web/20120501052352/http://www.thyroidmanager.o rg/chapter/acute-and-subacute-and-reidels-thyroiditis/ 2012*

Am J Clin Nutr 1980 33: 11 2338-45 "Lectins in the United States diet: a survey of lectins in commonly consumed foods and a review of the literature"

Amanda Hernandez "6 Essential Nutrients and Their Functions" Healthy Eating web Nov. 08, 2017

Amazing Discoveries. 2016. "The Eight Laws of Health." Accessed October 7.http://amazingdiscoveries.org/H-deception-health_laws_nutrition_exercise.

Ambooken Betsy, MP. Binitha and S. Sarita 2013 "Zinc Deficiency Associated with Hypothyroidism: An Overlooked Cause of Severe Alopecia" 2013 Jan-Mar; 5(1): 40–42. PMC web. Nov. 08, 2017

American Academy of Family Physicians. 2014. "Thyroiditis Overview," *FamilyDoctor.* Last modified May. http://familydoctor.org/familydoctor/en/diseases-conditions/thyroiditis.html.

American Association for Clinical Chemistry. 2016. "Thyroid Antibodies: The Test." Last modified September 21. https://labtestsonline.org/understanding/analytes/thyroid-antibodies/tab/test/.

American Autoimmune Related Diseases Association, Inc. 2016. "List of Diseases." Accessed October 7. https://www.aarda.org/autoimmune-information/list-of-diseases/.

—. 2016. "Questions and Answers." Accessed October 7. https://www.aarda.org/autoimmune-information/questions-and-answers/.

American Thyroid Association. 2016. "Thyroiditis." Accessed October 7. http://www.thyroid.org/thyroiditis/.

Anderson DM, Brydon WG, Eastwood MA, Sedwick DM. 1991 "Dietary effects of sodium alginate in humans." 1991 May-Jun;8(3):237-48. NCBI web Nov. 08, 2017

Appleby, Maia. 2016. "Recommended Levels of Essential Amino Acids," *SFGATE.* web. Nov. 08, 2017

Annals of clinical & laboratory science 2010
Green tea (Camelia sinensis) suppresses B cell production of IgE without inducing apoptosis.

Hassanain E, Silverberg JI, Norowitz KB, Chice S, Bluth MH, Brody N, Joks R, Durkin HG, Smith-Norowitz TA. http://www.annclinlabsci.org/content/40/2/135.long

Anderson, Jane. 2016. "Wheat Allergy vs. Gluten Allergy: Which Do You Have?" *Verywell.* Last modified May 5. https://www.verywell.com/what-are-gluten-allergy-symptoms-563120.

Dr. Andrew Weil "Why Bitter is Better" Huffington Post 04/28/2014 n. p. web oct. 24, 2017

Appleby, Maia. 2016. "Recommended Levels of Essential Amino Acids," *SFGATE*. Accessed October 7. http://healthyeating.sfgate.com/recommended-levels-essential-amino-acids-3649.html.

Arakawa, Y., Y. Hidaka, N. Inoue, Y. Iwatani, M. Sarumaru, and M. Watanabe. 2012. "Association of Polymorphisms in *DNMT1, DNMT3A, DNMT3B, MTHFR* and *MTRR* Genes with Global DNA Methylation Levels and Prognosis of Autoimmune Thyroid Disease," *Clinical & Experimental Immunology* 170(2) 194-201. doi: 10.1111/j.1365-2249.2012.04646.x.

ARJUN WALIA JULY 6, 2014 "19 SUPER FOODS THAT NATURALLY CLEANSE YOUR LIVER" Colective evolution web. Oct. 24, 2017 http://www.collective-evolution.com/2014/07/06/19-super-foods-that-naturally-cleanse-your-liver/

Aronson, Dina. 2009. "Cortisol — Its Role in Stress, Inflammation, and Indications for Diet Therapy," *Today's Dietitian* 11(11) page 38. http://www.todaysdietitian.com/newarchives/111609p38.shtml.

Arranz, E., D. Bernardo, L. Fernández-Salazar, J. A. Garrote, and S. Riestra. 2006. "Is Gliadin Really Safe for Non-Coeliac Individuals? Production of Interleukin 15 in Biopsy Culture from Non-Coeliac Individuals Challenged with Gliadin Peptides," *Gut* 2007 (56) 889-890. doi:10.1136/gut.2006.118265.

Arnarson, Atli. 2016. "6 Science-Based Health Benefits of Moringa Oleifera," *Authority Nutrition*. Accessed October 7. https://authoritynutrition.com/6-benefits-of-moringa-oleifera/.

Arthur JR, Nicol F, Beckett GJ. 1993 Feb. "Selenium deficiency, thyroid hormone metabolism, and thyroid hormone deiodinases." National Instite of Health web. October 15, 2017.

Asano, Masanao, Misako Itoh, Stephen S. Morse, Noriko Sakaguchi, Shimon Sakaguchi, and Masaaki Toda. 1996. "T Cell-Mediated Maintenance of Natural Self-Tolerance: Its Breakdown as a Possible Cause of Various Autoimmune Diseases," *Journal of Autoimmunity*, 9(2) 211-220. doi: 10.1006/jaut.1996.0026.

Atasoy, Ozgun. 2013. "Your Thoughts Can Release Abilities Beyond Normal Limits," *Scientific American*, August 13. https://www.scientificamerican.com/article/your-thoughts-can-release-abilities-beyond-normal-limits/.

Baba K., T. Fukaya, C. Mori, Y. Tomita, and M. Yoshizumi. 1978. "Computerized ECG Analysis in Cardiovascular Survey of Elementary-School Pupils," *Japanese Circulation Journal* 42(1) 53-6. https://www.ncbi.nlm.nih.gov/pubmed/633599.

Babal, Pavel, Pavol Janega, Andrea Janegova, Kristina Kuracinova, and Boris Rychly. 2015. "The Role of Epstein-Barr Virus Infection in the Development of Autoimmune Thyroid Diseases," *Endokrynologia Polska* 2015 66(2) 132-136. doi: 10.5603/EP.2015.0020.

Bart Deplancke and H Rex Gaskins 2001 "Microbial modulation of innate defense: goblet cells and the intestinal mucus layer" Am J Clin Nutr June 2001 vol. 73 no. 6 1131S-1141S web. Nov. 08, 2017

Bassett SM, Lupis SB, Gianferante D, Rohleder N, Wolf JM 2015 Sep 28. Sleep quality but not sleep quantity effects on cortisol responses to acute psychosocial stress. Web. Oct. 21, 2017

Bechtel, Jonathan. 2012. "Astragalus: It Stops Aging, Cancer, And More!" *Health Kismet*, July 13. http://blog.healthkismet.com/astragalus-health-benefits.

Bee Pollen Buzz. 2016. "Bee Pollen Dosage Recommendations." <http://www.bee-pollen-buzz.com/bee-pollen-dosage.html.> Accessed October 7, 2017

Beletate V, ElDib RP, Atallah AN. 2007 "Zinc supplementation for the prevention of type 2 diabetes mellitus." 2007 Jan 24;(1):CD005525. NCBI. Web Nov. 08, 2017

Beliefnet. 2016. "How to Control Your Mind and Thoughts." Accessed October 7. http://www.beliefnet.com/inspiration/ articles/how-to-control-your-mind-and-thoughts.aspx.

Bellipanni G, DI Marzo F, Blasi F, Di Marzo A. 2005 Dec;1057:393-402. "Effects of melatonin in perimenopausal and menopausal women: our personal experience." Web. Oct. 22, 2017.

Bennett, Jeanette M., Elizabeth J. Corwin, Laurence M. Demers, Laura Cousino Klein, Jan Ulbrecht, Kimberly N. Walter, and Courtney A. Whetzel. 2012. "Elevated Thyroid Stimulating Hormone Is Associated with Elevated Cortisol in Healthy Young Men and Women," *Thyroid Research* 5(13). doi: 10.1186/1756-6614-5-13.

Bensko, Tantra. 2009. "I Drink My Urine at You, Herr Doktore!" *Unlikely 2.0*, December 2009. http://www.unlikelystories.org/09/bensko1209.shtml.

Berk, Dottie, Lee S. Berk, and Stanley A. Tan. 2008. "Cortisol and Catecholamine Stress Hormone Decrease Is Associated With the Behavior of Perceptual Anticipation of Mirthful Laughter," *FASEB Journal* 22 946.11. http://www.fasebj.org/cgi/content/meeting_abstract/22/1_MeetingAbstracts/946.11.

Berry G.T., A.l. Coelho, and M.E. Rubio-Gozalbo. 2015. "Galactose Metabolism and Health," *Current Opinion in Clinical Nutrition and Metabolic Care* 18(4) 422-7. doi: 10.1097/MCO.0000000000000189.

Bès C., D. Bresson, N. Chapal, T. Chardès, V. Giudicelli, M.P. Lefranc, S. Péraldi-Roux. 2002. "The Human Anti-Thyroid Peroxidase Autoantibody Repertoire in Graves' and Hashimoto's Autoimmune Thyroid Diseases," *Immunogenetics* 54(3) 141-57. doi: 10.1007/s00251-002-0453-9.

BILL SCHOENBART AND ELLEN SHEFI " Organs Overview" How Stuff Works n d. n. p. web Oct. 24, 2017

Biology Notes with Questions & Answers. 2016. "What Is the Life Span of Antibodies in Body Circulation?" Accessed October 7. http://biotechnologyclass.blogspot.ca/2010/08/what-is-life-span-of-antibodies-in-body.html.

Biology of Belief. 2014. "What Thoughts and Emotions Are Affecting Your Cells? Here Is The Science Behind It.," August 28. https://biologyofbelief.wordpress.com/2014/08/28/what-thoughts-and-emotions-are-affecting-your-cells-here-is-the-science-behind-it/.

Biron, Christine A., Andrew H. Miller, Brad D. Pearce, and Marni N. Silverman. 2005. "Immune Modulation of the Hypothalamic-Pituitary-Adrenal (HPA) Axis During Viral Infection," *Viral Immunology* 18(1) 41-78. doi:10.1089/vim.2005.18.41.

Blannin, A. K., L. M. Castell, M. Gleeson, P. J. Robson, and N. P. Walsh. 1999. "Effects of Exercise Intensity, Duration and Recovery on in vitro Neutrophil Function in Male Athletes," *International Journal of Sports Medicine* 20(2) 128-130. doi: 10.1055/s-2007-971106.

Bluth, Martin H., Neil Brody, Seto Chice, Helen G. Durkin, Ehab Hassanain, Rauno Joks, Kevin B. Norowitz, Jonathan I. Silverberg, and Tamar A. Smith-Norowitz. 2010. "Green Tea (*Camelia sinensis*) Suppresses B Cell Production of IgE Without Inducing Apoptosis," *Annals of Clinical & Laboratory Science* 40 (2) 135-143. http://www.annclinlabsci.org/content/40/ 2/135.long.

Bollen M, Stalmans W. 1988 Jun "The effect of the thyroid status on the activation of glycogen synthase in liver cells." US National Library Medicine web. October 15, 2017

Boskey, Elizabeth and Carmella Wint. 2012. "Hashimoto's Disease," *Healthline*, August 16. http://www.healthline.com/health/ chronic-thyroiditis-hashimotos-disease.

Bosma, Anneleen and Claudia Mauri. 2012. "Immune Regulatory Function of B Cells," *Annual Review of Immunology* 30 221-241. doi: 10.1146/annurev-immunol-020711-074934.

Boundless. 2016. *Boundless Anatomy and Physiology. Types of Neurotransmitters by Function.* n.p.. https://www.boundless.com/physiology/textbooks/boundless-anatomy-and-physiology-textbook/overview-of-the-nervous-system-11/neurophysiology-113/types-of-neurotransmitters-by-function-619-3349/.

Breaking the vicious cycle. "D-manose" http://www.breakingtheviciouscycle.info/knowledge_base/detail/d-manose-in-fruit/

Breene, Sophia. 2013. "13 Unexpected Benefits of Exercise," *Greatist*, October 7. http://greatist.com/fitness/13-awesome-mental-health-benefits-exercise.

Brehar, Andreea, Alexandra Bulgar, Constantin Dumitrache, and Diana Paun. 2011. "MTHFR Mutations in Female Patients with Autoimmune Thyroiditis," *Endocrine Abstracts* (2011) 26 p110. http://www.endocrine-abstracts.org/ea/0026/ ea0026p110.htm.

Briden, Lara. 2013. "Why Thyroid Tests Are Unreliable," *Lara Briden's Healthy Hormone Blog*, April 5. http://www.larabriden.com/why-thyroid-tests-are-unreliable/.

Bright JJ. 2007 Curcumin and autoimmune disease. Turmeric for health Nov. 08, 2017

Buller, Amanda J., Carol S. Johnston, and Cindy M. Kim. 2004. "Vinegar Improves Insulin Sensitivity to a High-Carbohydrate Meal in Subjects with Insulin Resistance or Type 2 Diabetes," *Diabetes Care* 27 (1) 281-282. doi: 10.2337/diacare.27.1.281.

BusinessWire. 2016. "Antibodies Market to Grow at a CAGR of 12.5%: Global Industry Analysis and Opportunity Assessment 2016-2026 - Research and Markets," August 19. http://www.businesswire.com/news/home/20160819005230/en/Antibodies-Market-Grow-CAGR-12.5-Global-Indusrty.

Buxton O., G. Copinschi, R. Leproult, and E. Van Cauter. 1997. "Sleep Loss Results in an Elevation of Cortisol Levels the Next Evening," *Sleep* 20(10) 865-70. https://www.ncbi.nlm.nih.gov/pubmed/9415946.

Byron J. Richards, Board Certified Clinical Nutritionist "A Surprise Finding: Endothelial Cells Rejuvenate Your Liver" Wellness Resources Jan. 2011 n. d. n. p. web. Oct. 24, 2017.

C. Giuliani, MD, PHD, S. Di Santo, A. Hysi, M. Iezzi, MD, I. Bucci, M.D., G. Napolitano, MD April 3, 2016. University of Chieti-Pescara, Chieti, Italy. Medical advisor Journal. Web) October 14, 2017

Calabrese, Leonard H., Lelise Getu, Daniel M. Huck, Chris T. Longenecker, Grace Mirembe, Amy S. Nowacki, Emmy Okello, Robert A. Salata, Gregg J. Silverman, Isaac Ssinabulya, and David A. Zidar. 2016. "Role of Natural Autoantibodies in Ugandans With Rheumatic Heart Disease and HIV," *eBioMedicine* 2016 5 161-166. doi: 10.1016/j.ebiom.2016.02.006.

Callier, Viviane. 2016. "Autoimmune Diseases May Be Side Effect of a Strong Immune System," *New Scientist*, July 20. https://www.newscientist.com/article/2099313-autoimmune-diseases-may-be-side-effect-of-a-strong-immune-system/.

Cancer Survivors Network. 2011. "Can Thyroid Regenerate?" October 5. https://csn.cancer.org/node/227752.

Carnegie Mellon University. 2016. "How Stress Influences Disease: Study Reveals Inflammation as the Culprit," *ScienceDaily*. Accessed October 7. www.sciencedaily.com/releases/2012/04/120402162546.htm.

Carlos Mano. "Vegetables that contain salimarin" Healthy Living n. d. n.p. web. Oct. 24, 2017

Carroccio, Antonio, Carlo Catassi, Maria Grazia Clemente, Cinzia D'Agate, Mariarosaria Di Pierro, Sandro Drago, Ramzi El Asmar, Alessio Fasano, Giuseppe Iacono, Tarcisio Not, Amit Tripathi Anna Sapone, Manjusha Thakar, and Lucia Zampini. 2006. "Gliadin, Zonulin and Gut Permeability: Effects on Celiac and Non-Celiac Intestinal Mucosa and Intestinal Cell Lines," *Scandinavian Journal of Gastroenterology* 41(4) 408-419. doi: 10.1080/00365520500235334.

Casali, Paolo and Keith Elkon. 2008. "Nature and Functions of Autoantibodies," *Nature Reviews Rheumatology* 4, 491-498. doi: 10.1038/ncprheum0895.

Castro, Rosario, Samuel A.M. Martin, Christopher J. Secombes, and Jun Zou. 2011. "Cortisol Modulates the Induction of Inflammatory Gene Expression in a Rainbow Trout Macrophage Cell Line," *Fish & Shellfish Immunology* 30(1) 215-223. doi: 10.1016/j.fsi.2010.10.010.

Centre for Studies on Human Stress. 2016. "Acute vs. Chronic Stress." Accessed October 7. http://www.humanstress.ca/stress/ understand-your-stress/acute-vs-chronic-stress.html.

Chamberlin, Katy. 2009. "Exercise," *Amazing Discoveries*, April 6. http://amazingdiscoveries.org/H-deception-exercise_benefits_energy.

Chiara Dalla Pellegrina et al. "Effects_of_wheat_germ_agglutinin_on_human_gastroin" Research Gate DOI: 10.1016/j.taap.2009.03.012 n. page web. nov. 08, 2017

Chida Y, Sudo N. and Kubo C. Jan 2006. "Does stress exacerbate liver diseases?" National Institute of Health DOI:10.1111/j.1440-1746.2006.04110.x n. d. n. p. web. Oct. 24, 2017.

Chistiakov, Dimitry A. 2005. "Immunogenetics of Hashimoto's Thyroiditis," *Journal of Autoimmune Diseases* 2005 2(1). doi: 10.1186/1740-2557-2-1.

Chris Kresser "The Thyroid-Gut Connection" *JULY 29, 2010*

Chyun, Yong S., Barbara E. Kream, and Lawrence G. Raisz. 1984. "Cortisol Decreases Bone Formation by Inhibiting Periosteal Cell Proliferation," *Endocrinology* 114 (477). doi: 10.1210/endo-114-2-477.

City Allergy. 2016. "The Process of an Allergic Reaction." Accessed October 7. http://www.cityallergy.com/13-the-process-of-an-allergic-reaction/.

Cohen, Sheldon, William J. Doyle, Denise Janicki-Deverts, Gregory E. Miller, Ellen Frank, Bruce S. Rabine, and Ronald B. Turner. 2012. "Chronic Stress, Glucocorticoid Receptor Resistance, Inflammation, and Disease Risk," *Proceedings of the National Academy of Sciences* 109(16) 5995–5999. http://www.pnas.org/content/109/16/5995.

Commonly Prescribed Medications 2015 http://www.sdha.ca/wp-content/uploads/2014/10/Pharmacology-Handout-Dr.-Ann-Spolarich.pdf

Corazzaa, Gino Roberto, Paolo Giuffridaa, Antonio Di Sabatinoa, Ombretta Luinettib, Enrico Solciab, and Alessandro Vanolib. 2012. "The Function of Tissue Transglutaminase in Celiac Disease," *Autoimmunity Reviews* 11(10) 746–753. doi: 10.1016/j.autrev.2012.01.007

Creswell J Eastman, M.D. and Michael B Zimmermann, M.D updated July 2017 "The Iodine Deficiency Disorders" web. Oct. 16, 2017

D. Adamo. "DIABETES: THE LECTIN TRIGGER" Personalized Nutrition Jan. 2015 n. page. Web Nov. 08, 2017

D Bernardo, J A Garrote, L Fernández-Salazar, S Riestra. 2007 "Is gliadin really safe for non-coeliac individuals? Production of interleukin 15 in biopsy culture from non-coeliac individuals challenged with gliadin peptides." *Gut* 56.6 (2007): 889–890. *PMC*. Web. 8 Nov. 2017.

David Gutrierrez, Natural News, 2013 web. Oct. 16, 2017 David Peterson, DC, DCCN, FAAIM "The Genetically Modified Food Connection with Invisible Illness" Wellnes Alternative Jan. 2013 n. page. Web Nov. 08,2017 David Wolfe 2016https://www.davidwolfe.com/1-tablespoon-coconut-oil-day-thyroid/Eagleson C, Hayes S, Mathews A, Perman G, Hirsch CR. 2016 Mar.

D'Anci, Kristen E., Barry M. Popkin, and Irwin H. Rosenberg. 2010. "Water, Hydration, and Health," *Nutrition Reviews* 68(8): 439–458. doi: 10.1111/j.1753-4887.2010.00304.x.

Dairy Moos. 2013. "3 Reasons Why Lactose is Good for You," October 27. http://www.dairymoos.com/why-lactose-is-good-for-you/.

Dalmau, Josep and Matthew S. Kayser. 2010. "The Emerging Link Between Autoimmune Disorders and Neuropsychiatric Disease," *Journal of Neuropsychiatry and Clinical Neuroscience* 23(1) 90-97. http://neuro.psychiatryonline.org/doi/ full/10.1176/jnp.23.1.jnp90.

Dayan, C.M. and P. Saravanan. 2001. "Thyroid Autoantibodies," *Endocrinology and Metabolism Clinics of North America* 30(2) 315-37, viii. https://www.ncbi.nlm.nih.gov/pubmed/11444165.

Debbie Hampton, How thoughts change your cells and genes, 2016 http://www.huffingtonpost.com/debbie-hampton/how-your-thoughts-change-your-brain-cells-and-genes_b_9516176.html

DeLeve, Laurie D. "Liver Sinusoidal Endothelial Cells and Liver Regeneration." *The Journal of Clinical Investigation* 123.5 (2013): 1861–1866. *PMC*. Web. 8 Nov. 2017.

Dell DD and Kehoe C.1996. Plasma cholinesterase deficiency. 1996 Oct;11(5):304-8. NCBI n. page. Web Nov. 08, 2017https://www.ncbi.nlm.nih.gov/pubmed/8970294

Demehri, Afrouz. 2015. "Top Herbs for Hashimoto's," *AIM for Women*, August 5. http://www.aimforwomen.com/top-herbs-for-hashimotos/.

Desailloud, Rachel and Didier Hober. 2009. "Viruses and Thyroiditis: An Update," *Virology Journal* 2009 6(5). doi: 10.1186/1743-422X-6-5.

Deshpande UR, Joseph LJ, Patwardhan UN, Samuel AM. 2002 Jun;40(6):735-8. "Effect of antioxidants (vitamin C, E and turmeric extract) on methimazole induced hypothyroidism in rats." 2002 Jun;40(6):735-8. NCBI web Nov. 08, 2017

Diabetes information. "Niacinamide" <http://diabetesinformationhub.com/DiabetesNutrition_Niacinamide.php> n. d. n. page, web nov. 08, 2017

Dictionary.com Unabridged, s.v. 2016. "Autoimmune disease." Random House, Inc. Accessed October 7. http://www.dictionary.com/browse/autoimmune-disease.

Diego, Miguel, Tiffany Field, Maria Hernandez-Reif, Cynthia Kuhn, and Saul Schanberg. 2004. "Cortisol Decreases and Serotonin and Dopamine Increase Following Massage Therapy," *International Journal of Neuroscience* 115(10) 1397-1413. doi: 10.1080/00207450590956459.

Diet-and-Health.net. "Information on Histidine." Accessed October 7. http://www.diet-and-health.net/Supplements/ Histidine.html.

Dietitians of Canada http://www.dietitians.ca/Your-Health/Nutrition-A-Z/Fat/Food-Sources-of-Omega-3-Fats.aspx

Djurica S and B. Trbojević. 2005. "Diagnosis of Autoimmune Thyroid Disease [Article in Serbian]," *Srpski arhiv za celokupno lekarstvo* 133 Suppl 1:25-33. https://www.ncbi.nlm.nih.gov/pubmed/16405253.

Dohi, Toshihiro, Tomoya Kitayama, Norimitsu Morioka, Katsuya Morita, and Naoyo Motoyama. 2009. "Glycine Transporter Inhibitors as a Novel Drug Discovery Strategy for Neuropathic Pain," *Pharmacology & Therapeutics* 123(1) 54-79. doi: 10.1016/j.pharmthera.2009.03.018.

Dr. Atkins founder of the Atkins' Diet. "Zinc, Copper and Your Thyroid" Progresive health, web. Oct. 15, 2017

Dr. Axe. "20 Unique Apple Cider Vinegar Uses and Benefits" Food is Medicine n. d., n. p. web Oct.24, 2017

Dr. Axe. 2016. "Ashwagandha Benefits Thyroid and Adrenals." Accessed October 7. https://draxe.com/ashwagandha-proven-to-heal-thyroid-and-adrenals/.

—. 2016. "Balancing Act: Why pH is Crucial to Health." Accessed October 7. https://draxe.com/balancing-act-why-ph-is-crucial-to-health/.

—. 2016. "5 Natural Remedies for Thyroid Health." Accessed October 7. https://draxe.com/natural-remedies-for-thyroid/.

—. 2016. "9 Chia Seeds Benefits + Side Effects." Accessed October 7. https://draxe.com/chia-seeds-benefits-side-effects/.

Dr. Edward Group DC, NP, DACBN, DCBCN, DABFM "Liver Cleanse Food" Natural Health January 31, 2013, Global Healing Center. n. p. Web. Oct. 24, 2017

Dr. Izabella Wents farm D. http://thyroidpharmacist.com/articles/is-it-possible-to-recover-thyroid-function-in-hashimotos

Dr. Izabella Wentz Pharm D 2015 Tumeric for your thyroid and Hashimoto's http://thyroidpharmacist.com/articles/turmeric-for-your-thyroid-and-hashimotos/

Dr james L Wilson "Adrenal Fatigue" Web. Oct. 21, 2017

Dr Louis ignarro. "Why Focus on Endothelial Health?" n.d. n. p. web Oct.24, 2017 http://www.drignarro.com/why-focus-on-endothelial-health/

Dr. Mary Jane Brown, RD "How Short-Chain Fatty Acids Affect Health and Weight " Health line Authority Nutrition. April 2016. Web Nov. 08, 2017

Dr. Nikolas Hedberg, D.C., D.A.B.C.I., D.A.C.B.N. web. Oct.16, 2017

Dr. Peter Osborne 2015 " Dana Trentini10 Nutrient Deficiencies Every Thyroid Patient Should Have Checked" Hypothyroid mom. Web. Oct. 16, 2017

Dr. Weil.com. 2015. "Astragalus." Reviewed February. http://www.drweil.com/vitamins-supplements-herbs/herbs/astragalus/.

Drago S, El Asmar R, Di Pierro M, Grazia Clemente M, Tripathi A, Sapone A, Thakar M, Iacono G, Carroccio A, D'Agate C, Not T, Zampini L, Catassi C, Fasano A. 2006. "Gliadin, zonulin and gut permeability: Effects on celiac and non-celiac intestinal mucosa and intestinal cell lines." 2006 Apr;41(4):408-19. NCBI wb Nov. 08 2017

Duan H, Yuan Y, Zhang L, Qin S, Zhang K, Buchanan TW, Wu J. 2013 Nov. "Chronic stress exposure decreases the cortisol awakening response in healthy young men." Web. Oct. 21, 2017

Duke, J. A. CRC Handbook of Medicinal Herbs. Boca Raton, FL: CRC Press, 1985. Web. October 14, 2017

Ebert EC. 2010 "The thyroid and the gut." Web. Oct. 1,2017

Ede, Georgia. 2016. "Freshness Counts: Histamine Intolerance," Diagnosis: Diet. Accessed October 7. http://www.diagnosisdiet.com/histamine-intolerance/.

Educator – Sayer Ji. "Dangers of Wheat Germ Agglutinin (WGA)" Town Center Wellness n. page. Web. Nov. 08,2017 http://towncenterwellness.com/announcements/dangers-of-wheat-germ-agglutinin-wga

El Asmar R, Panigrahi P, Bamford P, Berti I, Not T, Coppa GV, Catassi C, Fasano A. "Host-dependent zonulin secretion causes the impairment of the small intestine barrier function after bacterial exposure." 2002 Nov;123(5):1607-15. NCBI web. Nov. 08, 2017

Elenkov, Ilia J. 2004. "Glucocorticoids and the Th1/Th2 Balance," Annals of the New York Academy of Sciences 1024 138-146. doi: 10.1196/annals.1321.010.

Elhomsy, Georges. 2014. "Antithyroid Antibody," Medscape. Last modified December 4. http://emedicine.medscape.com/ article/2086819-overview.

Elkin, Allen. 2016. "Thoughts That Cause Stress," Dummies.com. Accessed October 7. http://www.dummies.com/health/ mental-health/stress-management/thoughts-that-cause-stress/.

eLS. 2015. "Drosophila Oogenesis." John Wiley & Sons Ltd, Chichester. doi: 10.1002/9780470015902.a0001502.pub2.

Encyclopaedia Britanica Sucrose https://www.britannica.com/science/sucrose

ENDOCRINE SOCIETY
Thyroid Regeneration: Characterization of Clear Cells After Partial
Thyroidectomy" Takashi Ozaki, Tsutomu Matsubara, Daekwan Seo, Minoru
Okamoto, Kunio Nagashima, Yoshihito Sasaki, Suguru Hayase, Tsubasa
Murata, Xiao-Hui Liao, Jaime Rodriguez-Canales, Snorri S.
Thorgeirsson, Kennichi Kakudo, Samuel Refetoff, and   Kimura

ergo-log.com. 2016. "Fructose is a cortisol booster." Accessed October 7.
http://ergo-log.com/fructose-is-a-cortisol-booster.html.

Ertmann, M., E.F. Knol, A.C. Knulst, S.J. Koppelman, and M. Wensing. 2004.
"Relevance of Ara h1, Ara h2 and Ara h3 in Peanut-Allergic Patients, as
Determined by Immunoglobulin E Western Blotting, Basophil–Histamine
Release and Intracutaneous Testing: Ara h2 Is the Most Important Peanut
Allergen," *Clinical & Experimental Allergy* 34(4) 583–590.
doi:10.1111/j.1365-2222.2004.1923.x.

European Hydration Institute. 2016. "The Importance of Hydration." Last
modified June 14.
http://www.europeanhydrationinstitute.org/hydration.html.

Experience Life. 2010. "Drink to Your Health," June 2010.
https://experiencelife.com/article/drink-to-your-health/.

Faith R.E., D.N. Khansari, and A.J. Murgo. 1990. "Effects of Stress on the
Immune System," *Immunology Today* 11(5) 170-5.
https://www.ncbi.nlm.nih.gov/pubmed/2186751.

FAO. "toxic substances and antinutritional factors. Agriculture and Consumer
protection web. Oct. 16, 2017.

Farag, Noha H., William R. Lovallo, Terrie L. Thomas, Andrea S. Vincent, and
Michael F. Wilson. 2006. "Cortisol Responses to Mental Stress, Exercise,
and Meals Following Caffeine Intake in Men and Women," *Pharmacology
Biochemistry and Behavior* 83(3) 441-447. doi: 10.1016/j.pbb.2006.03.005.

Farhangi MA, Keshavarz SA, Eshraghian M, Ostadrahimi A, Saboor-Yaraghi
AA. 2012 Aug. "The effect of vitamin A supplementation on thyroid function
in premenopausal women." Web. Oct.15, 2017.

Fasano, Alessio, Anna Sapone, Detlef Schuppan, and Victor Zevallos. 2015.
"Nonceliac Gluten Sensitivity," *Gastroenterology* 148(6) 1195-1204. doi:
10.1053/j.gastro.2014.12.049.

Fawne Hansen "what are the adrenals" Adrenal fatigue solution. Web. Oct. 21, 2017

Felicetti, Marcus Julian. 2012. "How to Balance Your pH to Heal Your Body," *mindbodygreen*, September 24. http://www.mindbodygreen.com/0-6243/How-to-Balance-Your-pH-to-Heal-Your-Body.html.

Ferry, Robert Jr. 2016. "Hashimoto's Thyroiditis," *MedicineNet*. Last modified October 5. http://www.medicinenet.com/hashimotos_thyroiditis/page4.htm.

Fleckenstein, Burkhard, Günther Jung, Martin R. Larsen, Shuo-Wang Qiao, Peter Roepstorff, and Ludvig M. Sollid. 2004. "Molecular Characterization of Covalent Complexes between Tissue Transglutaminase and Gliadin Peptides," *The Journal of Biological Chemistry* 279, 17607-17616. doi: 10.1074/jbc.M310198200.

Food democracy 2013 "Wheat, gliadin, zonulin, auto immune, inflammation and you! Yes You!" Pual Cezanne jan 2013 web Nov. 08, 2017

Freed, David L J. "Do Dietary Lectins Cause Disease?: The Evidence Is Suggestive—and Raises Interesting Possibilities for Treatment." *BMJ: British Medical Journal* 318.7190 (1999): 1023–1024. Print.

Gaberšček, Simona and Katja Zaletel. 2011. "Hashimoto's Thyroiditis: From Genes to the Disease," *Current Genomics* 12(8) 576-588. doi: 10.2174/138920211798120763.

Gardner, Carol R., Debra L. Laskin, Jeffrey D. Laskin, and Vasanthi R. Sunil. 2011. "Macrophages and Tissue Injury: Agents of Defense or Destruction?" *Annual Review of Pharmacology and Toxicology* 51 267-288. doi: 10.1146/annurev.pharmtox.010909.105812.

Garnett Cheney 1949 "RAPID HEALING OF PEPTIC ULCERS IN PATIENTS RECEIVING FRESH CABBAGE JUICE" Wester Journal of medicine web oct. 24, 2017

Geiger AM, Pitts KP, Feldkamp J, Kirschbaum C, Wolf JM. 2015 Nov. "Cortisol-dependent stress effects on cell distribution in healthy individuals and individuals suffering from chronic adrenal insufficiency." Web. Oct. 21, 2017

GenScript. 2016. "Self-Tolerance." Accessed October 7. http://www.genscript.com/self-tolerance.html.

George Matelja Oct. 2017 "Cabbage" The World Healthiest foods. Web Oct. 24, 2017

Georgia Ede MD "Foods that cause hypothyroidism" Diagnosis Diet. Web. Oct. 22, 2017

Gerhard Uhlenbruck, PhD, MD "Eating right for your type" Dr. Peter D'Adamo and Catherine Whitney n. page. Web. nov. 08,2017

GIOVANNI BARBARA 2015 "Research finds new link between zonulin and 2 common inflammatory bowel conditions" Eurek Alert Oct 2015 web. Nov. 08, 2017

Glaser, Ronald and Janice K. Kiecolt-Glaser. 2005. "Stress-Induced Immune Dysfunction: Implications for Health," *Nature Reviews Immunology* 5, 243-251. doi: 10.1038/nri1571.

Glycobiology. Nathan Sharon Halina Lis History of lectins: from hemagglutinins to biological recognition molecules. Oxford Academy *Glycobiology*, Volume 14, Issue 11, 1 November 2004, Pages 53R–62R, web. Nov. 08,2017

GlyconutritionForLife. 2016. "Galactose." Accessed October 7. http://www.glyconutritionforlife.org/Science_of_ Glyconutrients/Galactose.php.

Goji berries. "What are goji berries?" 31 January 2007. HowStuffWorks.com. <https://recipes.howstuffworks.com/goji-berry.htm> 8 November 2017

Google search Thyriod hormone triggers the developmental loss of axonal regenerative capacity via thyroid hormone receptor α1 and krüppel-like factor 9 in Purkinje cells https://books.google.ca/books?id=u0KIC4bolb8C&pg=PA41&lpg=PA41&dq =thyroid+regeneration&source=bl&ots=-IsrqAJZfs&sig=HjT72pEy7DuOisi9a8ojf

Grammatikos, Alexandros P. and George C. Tsokos. 2012. "Immunodeficiency and Autoimmunity: Lessons from Systemic Lupus Erythematosus," *Trends in Molecular Medicine* 18(2) 101–108. doi: 10.1016/j.molmed.2011.10.005.

GreenMedinfo
6 Bodily Tissues That Can Be Regenerated Through Nutrition http://www.greenmedinfo.com/blog/6-bodily-tissues-can-be-regenerated-through-nutrition

Greer Fand Pusztai A. "Toxicity of kidney bean (Phaseolus vulgaris) in rats: changes in intestinal permeability." 1985;32(1):42-6 NCBI. N.page. web. Nov. 08,2017.

Greer MA. Goitrogenic substances in food. Am J Clin Nutr 1957; 5(4): 440-444. Nov. 08, 2017

Group, Edward. 2015. "3 Anti-Aging Benefits of Astragalus Root," *Global Healing Center*. Last modified February 27. http://www.globalhealingcenter.com/natural-health/3-ways-astragalus-root-promotes-youth-inside/.

Grönwall, Caroline and Gregg J. Sliverman. 2014. "Natural IgM: Beneficial Autoantibodies for the Control of Inflammatory and Autoimmune Disease?" *Journal of Clinical Immunology* 2014 34(1) 12-21. doi: 10.1007/s10875-014-0025-4.

Grönwall, Caroline, Gregg J. Sliverman, and Jaya Vas. 2012. "Protective Roles of Natural IgM Antibodies," *Frontiers in Immunology*. doi: 10.3389/fimmu.2012.00066.

Grumman Bender, Rachel. 2014. "People Are Drinking Vinegar. Should You?" *The Dr. Oz Show*, August 7. http://www.doctoroz.com/article/people-are-drinking-vinegar-should-you.

Gryalska E., Beata Matyjaszek-Matuszek, Aleksandra Pysik, and Jacek Rolinski. 2015. "Immune Disorders in Hashimoto's Thyroiditis: What Do We Know So Far?" *Journal of Immunology Research*. doi: 10.1155/2015/979167.

Gu-Jiun Lin, Shing-Hwa Huang, Shyi-Jou Chen, Chih-Hung Wang, Deh-Ming Chang, and Huey-Kang Sytwu 2013 May 31. "Modulation by Melatonin of the Pathogenesis of Inflammatory Autoimmune Diseases." Web. Oct 22, 2017.

Gunnars, Kris. 2016. "Daily Intake of Sugar – How Much Sugar Should You Eat Per Day?" *Authority Nutrition*. Accessed October 7. https://authoritynutrition.com/how-much-sugar-per-day/.

—. 2016. "How Much Water Should You Drink Per Day?" *Authority Nutrition*. Accessed October 7. https://authoritynutrition.com/how-much-water-should-you-drink-per-day/.

Hampton, Debbie. 2016. "How Your Thoughts Change Your Brain, Cells, And Genes," *The Best Brain Possible*. Accessed October 7. http://www.thebestbrainpossible.com/how-your-thoughts-change-your-brain-cells-and-genes/.

Hamilton, Jon. 2008. "Think You're Multitasking? Think Again," *NPR*, October 2. http://www.npr.org/templates/story/story.php?storyId=95256794.

Hampe, Christiane S. 2012. "B Cells in Autoimmune Diseases," *Scientifica* 2012. doi: 10.6064/2012/215308.

Hansen, Fawne. 2016. "Adrenal Fatigue and Your Immune System," *The Adrenal Fatigue Solution*. Accessed October 7. https://adrenalfatiguesolution.com/immune-system/.

Hanson, Jeffrey, Suguru Hayase, Kennichi Kakudo, Shioko Kimura, Xiao-Hui Liao, Tsutomu Matsubara, Tsubasa Murata, Kunio Nagashima, Minoru Okamoto, Takashi Ozaki, Samuel Refetoff, Jaime Rodriguez-Canales, Yoshihito Sasaki, Daekwan Seo, and Snorri S. Thorgeirsson. 2012. "Thyroid Regeneration: Characterization of Clear Cells After Partial Thyroidectomy," *Endocrinology* 153(5) 2514-2525. doi: 10.1210/en.2011-1365

Harriet Hall "Killer tomatoes poisonous potatoes" Science Based Medicine Feb 14, 2012. N. page web Nov. 08,2017

Harrison LC and Honeyman MC. "Cow's milk and type 1 diabetes: the real debate is about mucosal immune function." 1999 Aug;48(8):1501-7. NCBI n. page. Web. Nov. 08, 2017

Hashimoto's Healing. 2016. "Hashimoto's: How the Adrenals Cause All Kinds of Problems." Accessed October 7. https://www.hashimotoshealing.com/hashimotos-adrenals-cause-problems/.

Häussinger, Dieter. 1996. "The Role of Cellular Hydration in the Regulation of Cell Function," *Biochemical Journal* 313 (3) 697-710. doi: 10.1042/bj3130697.

Haymond, Morey W., Agneta Sunehag, and Stelios Tigas. 2002. "Contribution of Plasma Galactose and Glucose to Milk Lactose Synthesis during Galactose Ingestion," *The Journal of Clinical Endocrinology & Metabolism* 88 (1). doi: 10.1210/jc.2002-020768.

Health Alkaline. 2016. "4 Alkaline Minerals for pH Balance in Your Body." Accessed October 7. http://www.healthalkaline.com/4-alkaline-minerals-for-ph-balance-in-your-body/.

HealthAliciousNess. 2016. "Top 10 Foods Highest in Tryptophan." Last modified August 11. https://www.healthaliciousness.com/articles/high-tryptophan-foods.php.

Healthline. Caprilic acid 2016 http://www.healthline.com/health/caprylic-acid-coconut-oil#Benefits2

Hecht, Alan. 2008. *Mononucleosis (Deadly Diseases & Epidemics)*, 2nd ed. Chelsea House Publications.

Heikenwälder, Mathias. 2016. "Inflammation induced tissue damage," *VIRO*. Accessed October 7. https://www.helmholtz-muenchen.de/viro/research/working-groups/inflammation-induced-tissue-damage/research-focusfunding/index.html.

Hennessey, James V. 2011. "Riedel's Thyroiditis: A Clinical Review," *Journal of Clinical Endocrinology & Metabolism* 96(10). doi: 10.1210/jc.2011-0617.

Herb Wisdom http://www.herbwisdom.com/herb-bladderwrack.html

Heshmati J and Namazi N. 2015 "Effects of black seed (Nigella sativa) on metabolic parameters in diabetes mellitus: a systematic review." 2015 Apr;23(2):275-82. doi: 10.1016/j.ctim.2015.01.013. Epub 2015 Feb 9. NCBI n. page. Web. Nov. 08, 207

Heyma P, Larkins RG. 1982 Feb."Glucocorticoids decrease in conversion of thyroxine into 3, 5, 3'-tri-iodothyronine by isolated rat renal tubules." National Institute of Health. Web. October 15, 2017.

Hindawi Publishing Corporation
Curcumin Suppresses Metastasis via Sp-1, FAK Inhibition, and E-Cadherin Upregulation in Colorectal Cancer
https://www.hindawi.com/journals/ecam/2013/541695/

Histamine Intolerance. 2016. "The Food List." Accessed October 7. http://www.histamineintolerance.org.uk/about/the-food-diary/the-food-list/.

Holecek, Milan. 2010. "Three Targets of Branched-Chain Amino Acid Supplementation in the Treatment of Liver Disease," *Nutrition* 2(5) 482-90. doi: 10.1016/j.nut.2009.06.027.

Hood, Bruce. 2012. "Why Do We Need a Brain?" *Psychology Today*, April 30. https://www.psychologytoday.com/blog/ the-self-illusion/201204/why-do-we-need-brain.

Hopkins Autoimmune Disease Research Center. 2016. "What is Autoimmunity?" Accessed October 7. http://autoimmune.pathology.jhmi.edu/whatisautoimmunity.html.

HowtomakeX. 2016. "How to Reduce Cortisol," February 9. http://www.howtomakex.com/subject-how-to-reduce-cortisol.html.

Huang MJ, Liaw YF 1995 "Clinical associations between thyroid and liver diseases."

Hubert Kolb, Ph.D., Volker Burkart, Ph.D. "Nicotinamide in Type 1 Diabetes" Journal Diabetes n. page. N. d. web Nov. 08, 2017

Hughes, Katherine J., Ph.D., "Recovery of pancreatic beta-cells from nitric oxide-induced damage" Saint Louis University, ProQuest Dissertations Publishing, 2009. 338320 web. Nov. 08, 2017.

Hutchison, Kent E. and Robert L. Spencer. 1999. "Alcohol, Aging, and the Stress Response," *Alcohol Research & Health* 23(4). http://pubs.niaaa.nih.gov/publications/arh23-4/272-283.pdf.

H2O for Health. 2016. "How Acidity effects us." Accessed October 7. http://www.h2oforhealth.com/how-acidity-effects-us/.

Immune Deficiency Foundation, USA. 2016. "Autoimmunity." Accessed October 7. http://primaryimmune.org/about-primary-immunodeficiencies/relevant-info/autoimmunity/.

Indian J Psychiatry. 2009 The biochemistry of belief

   https://www.ncbi.nlm.nih.gov/pmc/articles/PMC2802367/

Innvista. 2011. "Galactose." Last modified June.
   http://innvista.com/health/nutrition/essential-sugars/galactose/.John

Israel today 2007
   Israelis link green tea to brain regeneration
   http://www.israeltoday.co.il/NewsItem/tabid/178/nid/14314/Default.aspx

J Med Food. 2008
   Immune modulation of macrophage pro-inflammatory response by goldenseal and Astragalus extracts.
   Clement-Kruzel S[1], Hwang SA, Kruzel MC, Dasgupta A, Actor JK.
   https://www.ncbi.nlm.nih.gov/pubmed/18800897

J Med Food. 2010 Zubeldia JM[1], Nabi HA, Jiménez del Río M, Genovese J. Exploring new applications for Rhodiola rosea: can we improve the quality of life of patients with short-term hypothyroidism induced by hormone withdrawal? https://www.ncbi.nlm.nih.gov/pubmed/20946017

Jabbar A, Yawar A, Waseem S, Islam N, Ul Haque N, Zuberi L, Khan A, Akhter J. 2008 May "Vitamin B12 deficiency common in primary hypothyroidism." NCBI. Web. Oct. 15, 2017.

Janet Renee Ms. RD "Is Honey Good for Your Liver?" Livestrong n. p. Aug. 14, 2017 web. Oct. 24, 2017 http://www.livestrong.com/article/478981-is-honey-good-for-your-liver/

Jaskanwal D. Sara, Ming Zhang, Hossein Gharib, Lilach O, Lerman, Amir Lerman July 2015. "Hypothyroidism ia Associated with Coronary Endothelial Dysfunction in Women" Journal of the American Heart Association. Web. Oct. 19, 2017

Jason Clark, BSc, MSc "What is nitric oxide and how does it work?" *nutrition express. n.page. web. Nov. 08, 2017*

Jawa A, Jawad A, Riaz SH, Assir MZ, Chaudhary AW, Zakria M, Akram J. 2015 May-Jun "Turmeric use is associated with reduced goitrogenesis: Thyroid disorder prevalence in Pakistan (THYPAK) study." 2015 May-Jun;19(3):347-50. doi: 10.4103/2230-8210.152768. NCBI web Nov. 08, 2017

Jeffers F, Fuell C, Tailford LE, Mackenzie DA, Bongaerts RJ, Juge N. Mucin-lectin interactions assessed by flow cytometry. 2010 Jul 2;345(10):1486-91. doi: 10.1016/j.carres.2010.05.012. Epub 2010 May 24 NCBI web. Nov. 08, 2017

JOHANNES MARTENSSON*, AJEY JAINt, AND ALTON MEISTER Proc. Natl. Acad. Sci. USA Vol. 87, pp. 1715-1719, March 1990 Biochemistry Glutathione is required for intestinal function.

Johnson, Richard J. and Robert Murray. 2010. "Fructose, Exercise, and Health," *Current Sports Medicine Reports* 9(4) 253-258. doi: 10.1249/JSR.0b013e3181e7def4.

JP. et al. 2009 "Lectins — A Little Known Trouble Maker" *The Institute for Natural Healing Jan 2009 n. page. Web Nov. 08, 2017*

Kar A., and S. Panda. 1998. "Changes in Thyroid Hormone Concentrations After Administration of Ashwagandha Root Extract to Adult Male Mice," *Journal of Pharmacy and Pharmacology* 50(9) 1065-8. Nov. 08, 2017

Kar, Anand and Pankaj Tahiliani. 2000. "Role of Moringa Oleifera Leaf Extract in the Regulation of Thyroid Hormone Status in Adult Male and Female Rats," *Pharmacological Research* 41 (3) 319-323. doi: 10.1006/phrs.1999.0587.

Katy Haldiman, MS, RN june 4 2013" The truth about stomach acid: Why low stomach acid is jeopardizing your health" The PALEO Nurse .web Oct. 24,2017

KidsHealth. 2015. "Immune System." Last modified May. http://m.kidshealth.org/en/parents/immune.html.

Kidd, Parris. 2003. "Th1/Th2 Balance: The Hypothesis, its Limitations, and Implications for Health and Disease," *Alternative Medicine Review* 8(3) 223-46. https://www.ncbi.nlm.nih.gov/pubmed/12946237.

Kim, Larry. 2015. "Multitasking Is Killing Your Brain," *Inc*, July 15. http://www.inc.com/larry-kim/why-multi-tasking-is-killing-your-brain.html.

Kim YH, Won YS, Yang X, Kumazoe M, Yamashita S, Hara A, Takagaki A, Goto K, Nanjo F, Tachibana H. "Green Tea Catechin Metabolites Exert Immunoregulatory Effects on CD4(+) T Cell and Natural Killer Cell Activities. 2016" 016 May 11;64(18):3591-7. doi: 10.1021/acs.jafc.6b01115. Epub 2016 May 2. NCBI web . Nov. 08, 2017

Kistler, Brandon M., Stephen A. Martin, Kenneth R. Wilund, and Jeffrey A. Woods. 2012. "Exercise, Inflammation and Aging," *Aging and Disease* 3(1) 130-140. https://www.ncbi.nlm.nih.gov/pmc/articles/PMC3320801/.

Kenichi Kitani 2007 Jan 11. doi: 10.1007/s11357-006-9014-8 "What really declines with age?" The Hayflick Lecture for 2006 35th American Aging Association. Web. Oct. 23, 2017.

Klein, John.R. 2006. "The Immune System as a Regulator of Thyroid Hormone Activity," *Experimental Biology and Medicine (Maywood, N.J.)* 231(3) 229-36. https://www.ncbi.nlm.nih.gov/pmc/articles/PMC2768616/.

Klein AV and Kiat H. 2015 "Detox diets for toxin elimination and weight management: a critical review of the evidence." National Institute of health n.p. web. Oct. 24, 2017

Klein, John.R. and H.C. Wang. 2001. "Immune Function of Thyroid Stimulating Hormone and Receptor," *Critical Reviews in Immunology* 21(4) 323-37. https://www.ncbi.nlm.nih.gov/pubmed/11922077.

Koyuncu A, Aydintu S, Koçak S, Aydin C, Demirer S, Topçu O, Kuterdem E. 2002 "Effect of thyroid hormones on stress ulcer formation." Web. Oct. 22, 2017

Krispin Sullivan, CN 10/05/16 THE LECTIN REPORT n. page web. Nov. 8, 17 Vasconcelos IM and Oliveira JT. 2004 " Antinut

Kronenberg, Henry M., P. Reed Larsen, Shlomo Melmed, and Kenneth S. Polonsky. 2011. *Williams Textbook of Endocrinology*, 12th ed. Philadelphia: Saunders.

Krull, Erika. 2016. "Depression and Letting Go of Negative Thoughts," *Psych Central*, July 17. http://psychcentral.com/lib/ depression-and-letting-go-of-negative-thoughts/.

Lai HS, Lin WH, Chen PR, Wu HC, Lee PH, Chen WJ. Nov. 2005 "Effects of a high-fiber diet on hepatocyte apoptosis and liver regeneration after partial hepatectomy in rats with fatty liver." National Institute of Health n. p. web Oct. 24, 2017

Lajolo FM and Genovese MI 2002 "Nutritional significance of lectins and enzyme inhibitors from legumes." 2002 Oct 23;50(22):6592-8 NCBI. N. page. Web Nov. 08,2017

LARRY ARMSTRONG "Vitamin B Complex & Diabetes" Live strong cot. 2013 web n. pagem web Nov. 08, 2017

Laskin, Debra L. and Kimberly J. Pendino. 1995. "Macrophages and Inflammatory Mediators in Tissue Injury," *Annual Review of Pharmacology and Toxicology* 35:655-677. doi: 10.1146/annurev.pa.35.040195.003255.

Leaf, Caroline. 2011. "You are What you Think: 75-98% of Mental and Physical Illnesses Come from our Thought Life!" *Dr. Leaf*, November 30. http://drleaf.com/blog/you-are-what-you-think-75-98-of-mental-and-physical-illnesses-come-from-our-thought-life/.

Leech, Joe. 2016. "10 Evidence-Based Health Benefits of Cinnamon," *Authority Nutrition*.. <https://authoritynutrition.com/10-proven-benefits-of-cinnamon/>. Web Accessed October 7, 2017

Lejuwaan, Jordan. 2016. "How Your Thoughts Program Your Cells," *High Existence*. Accessed October 7. http://highexistence.com/thoughts-program-cells/.

Li Y, Schellhorn HE 2007 "New developments and novel therapeutic perspectives for vitamin C." 007 Oct;137(10):2171-84. NCBI web. nov. 08, 2017

Life force international. Eight essential sugars http://www.liquidhealthproducts.com/eight-essential-sugars.htm

Lippi G, Montagnana M, Targher G, Salvagno GL, Guidi GC. 2008 Jul."Prevalence of folic Acid and vitamin B12 deficiencies in patients with thyroid disorders." NCBI. Web Oct. 15, 2017.

Liu IM, Liou SS, Lan TW, Hsu FL, Cheng JT "Myricetin as the active principle of Abelmoschus moschatus to lower plasma glucose in streptozotocin-induced diabetic rats." 2005 Jul;71(7):617-21. NCGI web. Nov. 08, 2017

Liu WK, Sze SC, Ho JC, Liu BP, Yu MC. 2004 "Wheat germ lectin induces G2/M arrest in mouse L929 fibroblasts." 2004 Apr 15;91(6):1159-73.NCBI web. Nov. 08,2017

Liver.ca Canadan liver Foundation Health Online web. Sept. 22, 2016

Livestrong, benefits of capric acid 2015
http://www.livestrong.com/article/475060-benefits-of-capric-acid/

Lüthy J, Carden B, Friederich U, Bachmann M (May 1984). "Goitrin--a nitrosatable constituent of plant foodstuffs". Experientia. **40** (5): 452–3. PMID 6723906. doi:10.1007/BF01952381. Web Nov. 08, 2017

MacMillan, Amanda. 2016. "5 Ways to Stop Dwelling on Negative Thoughts," *Happify*. Accessed October 7. http://www.happify.com/hd/stop-dwelling-on-negative-thoughts/.

Mahla, Ranjeet Singh. 2015. Comment in "Cleanup Crew," *Science* 347(6226) 1058-1061, March 6. http://www.comments.sciencemag.org/content/10.1126/science.347.6226.1058.

Maintz, Laura and Natalija Novak. 2007. "Histamine and Histamine Intolerance," *American Journal of Clinical Nutrition* 85(5) 1185-1196. http://ajcn.nutrition.org/content/85/5/1185.long.

Mandal, Ananya. 2014. "Low-Level Autoimmunity," *News-Medical.Net*. Last modified October 9. http://www.news-medical.net/health/Low-Level-Autoimmunity.aspx.

—. 2014. "What is Histamine?" *News-Medical.Net*. Last modified August 19. http://www.news-medical.net/health/what-is-histamine.aspx.

Mandel KG, Daggy BP, Brodie DA, Jacoby HI. 2000 "Review article: alginate-raft formulations in the treatment of heartburn and acid reflux." 2000 Jun;14(6):669-90. NCBI web Nov. 08, 2017

Manzoor, Mohammad. 2012. "Chronic Inflammation," *SlideShare*, December 30. http://www.slideshare.net/ drmohammadmanzoor/chronic-inflammation.

Marano, Hara Estroff. 2016. "Depression Doing the Thinking," *Psychology Today*. Last modified June 3https://www.psychologytoday.com/articles/200107/depression-doing-the-thinking.

Mark Hyman MD is the Director of Cleveland Clinic's Center for Functional Medicine, The Ultra Wellness Center, What is Glutathione and How Do I Get More of It? Web. Oct. 23, 2017.

Masahiro Okouchi, Naotsuka Okayama, and Tak Yee Aw[*] 2009 Nov; 6(4): 267–278. "Preservation of Cellular Glutathione Status and Mitochondrial Membrane Potential by N-Acetylcysteine and Insulin Sensitizers Prevent Carbonyl Stress-Induced Human Brain Endothelial Cell Apoptosis" web. Oct. 23,2017

Matcha Source. 2016. "Health Benefits of Matcha Tea." Accessed October 7. http://matchasource.com/health-benefits-of-matcha-tea/.

Mayo Clinic Staff. 2014. "Hashimoto's Disease Causes," *Mayo Clinic*, January 2. http://www.mayoclinic.org/diseases-conditions/hashimotos-disease/basics/causes/con-20030293.

—. 2014. "Hashimoto's Disease Definition," *Mayo Clinic*, January 2. http://www. mayoclinic.org/diseases-conditions/hashimotos-disease/basics/definition/con-20030293.

—. 2014. "Hashimoto's Disease Tests and Diagnosis," *Mayo Clinic*, January 2. http://www.mayoclinic.org/diseases-conditions/hashimotos-disease/basics/tests-diagnosis/con-20030293.

Mercola. Bee pollen as superfood. 2016 http://www.mercola.com/article/diet/bee_pollen.htm

Mercola, Joseph. 2008. "How Your Thoughts Can Cause or Cure Cancer," *Mercola.com*, February 19. http://articles.mercola.com/sites/articles/archive/2008/02/19/how-your-thoughts-can-cause-or-cure-cancer.aspx.

—. 2015. "How Apple Cider Vinegar Can Change Your Life," *Mercola.com*, March 21. http://articles.mercola.com/sites/articles/archive/2015/03/21/apple-cider-vinegar-uses.aspx.

—. "The Use of Bee Pollen as a Superfood," *Mercola.com*. Accessed October 7. http://www.mercola.com/article/diet/bee_pollen.htm.

McCoy, Krisha. 2015. "Understanding Autoimmunity," *Everyday Health*. Last modified December 21. http://www.everydayhealth.com/autoimmune-disorders/index.aspx.

McCraty, Rollin and Glen Rein. 2001. "Local and Non-Local Effects of Coherent Heart Frequencies on Conformational Changes of DNA," *HeartMath*. https://appreciativeinquiry.case.edu/practice/organizationDetail.cfm?coid=852&sector=2.

McDermott, Michael F. and Dennis McGonagle. 2006. "A Proposed Classification of the Immunological Diseases," *PLOS Medicine*. doi: 10.1371/journal.pmed.0030297.

McEvoy, Michael. 2011. "Acid & Alkaline Nutrition: Shattering the Myths," *Metabolic Healing*, December 12. https://metabolichealing.com/acid-alkaline-nutrition-shattering-the-myths/.

McGehee DS, Krasowski MD, Fung DL, Wilson B, Gronert GA, Moss J. Cholinesterase inhibition by potato glycoalkaloids slows mivacurium metabolism. PubMeb 2000 Aug;93(2):510-9. N. page web Nov. 08, 2017

MedicineNet.com. 2016. "Definition of Autoimmunity." Last modified May 13. http://www.medicinenet.com/script/ main/art.asp?articlekey=18985.

—. 2016. "Definition of Cytokine." Last modified May 13. http://www.medicinenet.com/script/main/ art.asp?articlekey=11937.

MedlinePlus. 2015. "Autoimmune Disorders." Last modified April 30. https://www.medlineplus.gov/ency/article/000816.htm.

—. 2016. "Hypothyroidism." Last modified March 20. https://medlineplus.gov/ency/article/000353.htm.

—. 2016. "Immune Response." Last modified March 20. https://medlineplus.gov/ency/article/000821.htm.

—. 2016. "Subacute Thyroiditis." Last modified February 3. https://medlineplus.gov/ency/article/000375.htm.

Merely Me. 2010. "Rhodiola Rosea to Treat Anxiety and Depression," *HealthCentral*, September 28. http://www.healthcentral.com/anxiety/c/849319/120854/rosea-depression/.

Meridian Health Clinic – Acupuncture & Chinese Herbal Medicine. Web Oct. 22,2017

Merriam-Webster, s.v. 2016. "Innate Immunity Medical Definition." Accessed October 7. http://www.merriam-webster.com/medical/innate%20immunity.

—. 2016. "Mind." Accessed October 7. http://www.merriam-webster.com/dictionary/mind.

—. 2016. "Nocebo." Accessed October 7. http://www.merriam-webster.com/dictionary/ nocebo.

Metcalfe, Dean D., Calman Prussin, and Kelly D. Stone. 2010. "IgE, Mast Cells, Basophils, and Eosinophils," *Journal of Allergy and Clinical Immunology* 125(2) Supplement 2 S73–S80. doi: 10.1016/j.jaci.2009.11.017.

Michael Edwards "Foods and supplements to heal your thyroid" Natural News, March 11, 2015. web. Oct.16, 2017.

Microbiology and Immunology On-line, University of South Carolina School of Medicine. 2016. "Immunology." Accessed October 7. http://www.microbiologybook.org/book/immunol-sta.htm.

Mike Barrett February. 11, 2013. "6 HEALTH BENEFITS OS OKRA" NATURAL SOCIETY WEB. OCT. 19. 1017

Mikkat U, Damm I, Schröder G, Schmidt K, Wirth C, Weber H, Jonas L. "Effect of the lectins wheat germ agglutinin (WGA) and Ulex europaeus agglutinin (UEA-I) on the alpha-amylase secretion of rat pancreas in vitro and in vivo". 1998 May;16(4):529-38. NCBI n. page web. Nov. 08,2017

Milas, Kresimira (Mira). 2014. "Causes of Hashimoto's Thyroiditis," *Endocrine Web*. Last modified May 29. http://www.endocrineweb.com/conditions/hashimotos-thyroiditis/causes-hashimotos-thyroiditis.

—. 2016. "Hashimoto's Thyroiditis Overview," *Endocrine Web*. Last   modified July 26. http://www.endocrineweb.com/conditions/hashimotos-oiditis/hashimotos-thyroiditis-overview

Modern Wheat is Bad For You 2016 http://intentionalwellnessinc.com/scoop-it/soy-deception/

Morris MC, Rao U. 2014 Jan "Cortisol response to psychosocial stress during a depressive episode and remission." Web. Oct. 21, 2017

Mountain State Centers for Independent Living. 2016. "What Is Stress?" Accessed October 7. http://www.mtstcil.org/skills/stress-definition-1.html.

Nadolsky, Karl. 2014. "Does Gluten Really Destroy Your Thyroid?," *Docs Who Lift*, January 5. http://docswholift.com/does-gluten-really-destroy-your-thyroid/.

Nafiseh Khandouzi, Farzad Shidfar, Asadollah Rajab, Tayebeh Rahideh, Payam Hosseini, and Mohsen Mir Taheri 2015 "The Effects of Ginger on Fasting Blood Sugar, Hemoglobin A1c, Apolipoprotein B, Apolipoprotein A-I and Malondialdehyde in Type 2 Diabetic Patients" Rahat Ali Khan, Trivendra Tripathi - 2010

Biomedical Aspects of Histamine: Current Perspectives Google books page 161 Nov. 08, 2017

Naomi Parker January 23, 2015 "To be or not to be." Web. Oct. 15, 2017

National Center for Complementary and Integrative Health. 2016. "Astragalus." Last modified January 5. https://nccih.nih.gov/health/astragalus.

National Health Service. 2015. "Benefits of Exercise." Last modified July 13. http://www.nhs.uk/livewell/fitness/Pages/ Whybeactive.aspx.

National Sleep Foundation. 2016. "Lights Out for a Good Night's Sleep." Accessed October 7. https://sleepfoundation.org/ sleep-news/lights-out-good-nights-sleep.

National sleep foundation 2016 https://sleepfoundation.org/sleep-topics/sleep-related-problems/allergic-rhinitis-and-sleep

NCBI 2016
CD24 molecule [Homo sapiens (human)]
https://www.ncbi.nlm.nih.gov/gene/100133941

New York Times. 2016. "Hypothyroidism In-Depth Report." Accessed October 7. http://www.nytimes.com/health/ guides/disease/hypothyroidism/print.html.

News medical life science 2008 "Findings reveal further detail about protein linked to inflammatory disorders" http://www.news-medical.net/news/20090908/Scientists-solve-the-mystery-of-zonulins-identity.aspx

Nicholas J. Mantis, PhD, Nicolas Rol, MSc, and Blaise Corthésy, PhD 2011 "Secretory IgA's Complex Roles in Immunity and Mucosal Homeostasis in the Gut" .2011 Nov; 4(6): 603–611. PMC werb. Nov. 08, 2017

Nippoldt, Todd B. 2015. "Thyroid peroxidase antibody test: What is it?" Mayo Clinic, June 17. http://www.mayoclinic.org/thyroid-disease/expert-answers/faq-20058114.

Noah ND, Bender AE, Reaidi GB, Gilbert RJ. "Food poisoning from raw red kidney beans." 1980 Jul 19;281(6234):236-7. NCBI n. page. Web. Nov. 08, 2017

Nordqvist, Christian. 2015. "Inflammation: Causes, Symptoms and Treatment," Medical News Today. Last modified September 16. http://www.medicalnewstoday.com/articles/248423.php.

Norman, James. 2016. "Hypothyroidism: Too Little Thyroid Hormone," *Endocrine Web*. Last modified April 11. http://www.endocrineweb.com/conditions/thyroid/hypothyroidism-too-little-thyroid-hormone.

Novimmune. 2016. "Antibodies." Accessed October 7. http://novimmune.com/science/antibodies.html.

Nussey S.S. and S.A. Whitehead. 2001. *Endocrinology: An Integrated Approach*. Oxford: BIOS Scientific Publishers.

Nutrientreviews.com. 2016. "Galactose." Accessed October 7. http://www.nutrientsreview.com/carbs/monosaccharides-galactose.html.

Nutrition and you "Okra nutrition facts" http://www.nutrition-and-you.com/okra.html

Nutritional-Supplements-Health-Guide.com. 2016. "L-Tyrosine Dosage - Can You Take Too Much L-tyrosine?" Accessed October 7. http://www.nutritional-supplements-health-guide.com/l-tyrosine-dosage.html.

Nutrition to Wellness. 2016. "What Are Essential Sugars and Why Are They Essential?" Accessed October 7. http://nutrition-now.com/2010/04/what-are-essential-sugars-and-why-are-they-essential/.

Oh S, Tanaka K, Warabi E, Shoda J. Dec. 2013 "Exercise reduces inflammation and oxidative stress in obesity-related liver diseases." National Institute of Health DOI:10.1249/MSS.0b013e31829afc33 n. d. n. p. web Oct. 24, 2017

Ooi LS, Li Y, Kam SL, Wang H, Wong EY, Ooi VE. "Antimicrobial activities of cinnamon oil and cinnamaldehyde from the Chinese medicinal herb Cinnamomum cassia Blume." 2006;34(3):51122. NCBI n.web. Nov. 08,

Ostman E, et al., "Vinegar supplementation lowers glucose and insulin responses and increases satiety after a bread meal in healthy subjects." National Institute of Medicine Sept. 2005 n. p. web Oct. 24, 2017

Paleo Leap. 2016. "All About Histamines." Accessed October 7. http://paleoleap.com/histamines/.

—. 2016. "Meet Your Thyroid: A Paleo Introduction." Accessed October 7. http://paleoleap.com/thyroid-a-paleo-introduction/.

Palacios, R. and I. Sugawara. 1982. "Hydrocortisone Abrogates Proliferation of T Cells in Autologous Mixed Lymphocyte Reaction by Rendering the Interleukin-2 Producer T Cells Unresponsive to Interleukin-1 and Unable to Synthesize the T-Cell Growth Factor," *Scandinavian Journal of Immunology* 15(1) 25-31. https://www.ncbi.nlm.nih.gov/pubmed/6461917.

Patel, Arti. 2015. "Goji Berry Benefits: 12 Facts About This Healthy Superfood," *Huffington Post Canada*. Last modified November 17. http://www.huffingtonpost.ca/2014/03/28/goji-berry-benefits-_n_5044948.html.

Pietro Ghezzi. 2011 Jan 25. doi: 10.2147/IJGM.S15618 "Role of glutathione in immunity and inflammation in the lung" Journal of General Medicine" web. Oct. 23,2017

PMC frontier in endocrinology
Thyroid Regeneration: How Stem Cells Play a Role?
https://www.ncbi.nlm.nih.gov/pmc/articles/PMC3995070/

Post-White J, Ladas EJ, Kelly KM. June 2007 "Advances in the use of milk thistle (Silybum marianum)." National Institute of Health DOI:10.1177/1534735407301632 n. d. n. p. web. Oct. 24, 2017

Proceedings of national academy of science of the United States of America. Thyroid hormone triggers the developmental loss of axonal regenerative capacity via thyroid hormone receptor α1 and krüppel-like factor 9 in Purkinje cells
http://www.pnas.org/content/109/35/14206.full

Poletaev, Alexander. 2014. "The Natural Autoimmunity: Self-Recognition, Self-Interaction, and Self-Maintenance," *Journal of Autoimmunity and Research*, July 19. https://www.jscimedcentral.com/Autoimmunity/autoimmunity-1-1001.php.

Psychology Today. 2016. "Mindfulness." Accessed October 7. https://www.psychologytoday.com/basics/mindfulness.

Pubmed health "How does the liver work?" US National Library of Medicine August 22, 2016 web. Oct. 24, 2017
https://www.ncbi.nlm.nih.gov/pubmedhealth/PMH0072577/

PubMed.gov Compensatory thyroid hypertrophy after hemithyroidectomy in rats.Clark OH, Lambert WR, Cavalieri RR, Rapoport B, Hammond ME, Ingbar SH.Biochemical and histological observations indicated that enlargement of the residual lobe was due to hypertrophy rather than hyperplasia. https://www.ncbi.nlm.nih.gov/pubmed/976198

PubMed.gov. thyroiditis: role of CD24.   Chen CY[1], Kimura H, Landek-Salgado MA, Hagedorn J, Kimura M, Suzuki K, Westra W, Rose NR, Caturegli P https://www.ncbi.nlm.nih.gov/pubmed/18801910

Pubmed.gov 2010 Effect of different doses of un-fractionated green and black tea extracts on thyroid physiology. Chandra AK, De N, Choudhury SR. https://www.ncbi.nlm.nih.gov/pubmed/20801949

Pure Healing Foods. 2016. "Hemp Seeds." Accessed October 7. http://www.purehealingfoods.com/hempHeartsInfo.php.

Putnam, David F. 1971. "Composition and Concentrative Properties of Human Urine," NASA Contractor Report, July 1971. http://ntrs.nasa.gov/archive/nasa/casi.ntrs.nasa.gov/19710023044.pdf.

Pusztai A. "Dietary lectins are metabolic signals for the gut and modulate immune and hormone functions." 1993 Oct;47(10):691-9. NCBI n. page. web. Nov.08,2017.

Quintana, Francisco J. and Howard L. Weiner. 2006. "Understanding Natural and Pathological Autoimmunity," *Journal of Neuroimmunology* 174 (2006) 1-2. web Oct. 10 2016

RadhaKrishna Rao and Geetha Samak "Role of Glutamine in Protection of Intestinal Epithelial Tight Junctions" 2012 Jan; 5(Suppl 1-M7): 47–54. PMC> web. web Nov. 08, 2017

Rafsanjani FN, Z Asl S, Naseri MK, Vahedian J. 2003 "Effects of thyroid hormones on basal and stimulated gastric acid secretion due to histamine, carbachol and pentagastrin in rats." Web. Oct. 19, 2017

Rana SV, Pal R, Vaiphei K, Singh K. 2006 "Garlic hepatotoxicity: safe dose of garlic." National Institute of Health. Web. Oct. 24, 2017 https://www.ncbi.nlm.nih.gov/pubmed/16910057

Ray Peat, PhD. 2005 "Benefits of the Raw Carrot" Functional Performance System. Web. October 15, 2017

Reasoner, Jordan. 2013. "Why Cortisol Is Good For You," *SCD Lifestyle*, October. http://scdlifestyle.com/2013/10/why-cortisol-is-good-for-you.

Robin Meywes Break through health diet and longevity clinic Jan 2010 web Nov. 08, 2017

Robinson, Lawrence, Jeanne Segal, Robert Segal, and Melinda Smith. 2016. "Stress Symptoms, Signs, and Causes," *HelpGuide.org*. Last modified October. http://www.helpguide.org/articles/stress/stress-symptoms-causes-and-effects.htm.

Roddick, Julie. 2015. "Autoimmune Disease," *Healthline*. Last modified July 22. http://www.healthline.com/health/ autoimmune-disorders.

Roos, Annemieke, et. al. "Thyroid Function Is Associated with Components of the Metabolic Syndrome in Euthyroid Subjects," *The Journal of Clinical Endocrinology & Metabolism* Vol. 92, No. 2 491-496, web. Oct. 15, 2017

Ruscio, Michael. 2016. "Inflammation – The Silent Thyroid Disruptor," *Primal Docs*. Accessed October 7. http://primaldocs.com/members-blog/inflammation-the-silent-thyroid-disruptor/.

Russian Breakthrough Unravels BCM7 Mysteries. Keith Woodford 2010. Lincoln University New Zealand n.page. web. Nov. 08,

Ryan Andrews "All about lectins" Precidion Nutrition n. page web. Nov. 08, 2017

S. La VigneraEmail author, R. Condorelli, E. Vicari, A. E. Calogero. January 2012, Volume 35, Issue 1, pp 96–103| Cite as "Endothelial dysfunction and subclinical hypothyroidism: A brief review" acesed Oct. 18, 2017.

Sahlin, K. 1986. "Muscle Fatigue and Lactic Acid Accumulation," *Acta Physiologica Scandinavia Supplementum* 1986;556:83-91. https://www.ncbi.nlm.nih.gov/pubmed/3471061.

Sakamoto S, Nakamura K, Inoue K, Sakai T. 2000 Sept "Melatonin stimulates thyroid-stimulating hormone accumulation in the thyrotropes of the rat pars tuberalis." Web. Oct. 22, 2017.

Santevia. 2016. "Why pH Balance." Accessed October 7. https://santevia.com/ph/.

Saraswati, Swami Shankardev and Jayne Stevenson. 2013. "Do You Think Too Much? What Neuroscientists and Yogis Say," *Big Shakti*, September 25. https://www.bigshakti.com/do-you-think-too-much/.

Sarich, Christina. 2013. "Achieving Alkalinity To Treat Illness And Disease: Changing Your PH Balance," *Natural Society*, August 25. http://naturalsociety.com/alkalinity-treat-disease-change-ph-balance/.

Sasson, Remez. 2016. "The Restless Mind - The Constantly Thinking Mind," *SuccessConsciousness.com.* Accessed October 7. http://www.successconsciousness.com/index_00007d.htm.

Sayer Ji, Founder "6 Bodily Tissues That Can Be Regenerated Through Nutrition" GreenMedInfo LLC, 2013 29th 2012 web. Nov. 08,2017

Schultz, Rachael. 2013. "The Worst Thing You Do Before Bed," *Men's Health*, September 18. http://www.menshealth.com/ health/the-worst-thing-you-do-before-bed.

Science direct 2004   A study on the immune receptors for polysaccharides from the roots of Astragalus membranaceus, a Chinese medicinal herb
Bao-Mei Shao,a Wen Xu,a Hui Dai,a Pengfei Tu,b Zhongjun Li,c and Xiao-Ming Gaoa
https://www.cap-tb.org/sites/default/files/documents/Astragalus.immunereceptors.pdf

Shoenfeld Yehuda and Y. Tomer. 1988. "The Significance of Natural Autoantibodies," *Immunological Investigations* 17(5) 389-424. https://www.ncbi.nlm.nih.gov/pubmed/3058585.

Shoenfeld, Yehuda and Elias Toubi. 2005. "Protective autoantibodies: role in homeostasis, clinical importance, and therapeutic potential," *Arthritis and Rheumatism*, vol. 52, no. 9, pp. 2599–2606.

Sietze Reitsma, Dick W. Slaaf, Hans Vink, Marc A. M. J. van Zandvoort, and Mirjam G. A. oude Egbrink 2007 "The endothelial glycocalyx: composition, functions, and visualization" *Pflugers Archiv* 454.3 (2007): 345–359. *PMC*. Web. 8 Nov. 2017.

Silberner, Joanne. 2010. "100 Years Ago, Exercise Was Blended Into Daily Life," *NPR*, June 7. http://www.npr.org/templates/story/story.php?storyId=127525702

Sollid LM, Kolberg J, Scott H, Ek J, Fausa O, Brandtzaeg P. 1986 "Antibodies to wheat germ agglutinin in coeliac disease." *Clinical and Experimental Immunology* 63.1 (1986): 95–100. Print.

.Speiser, Phyllis W. 2016. "Pediatric Adrenal Insufficiency (Addison Disease)," *Medscape*. Last modified June 19. http://emedicine.medscape.com/article/919077-overview.

Springer Link
Regeneration of the thyroid gland (study)1963
R. A. Gibadulin
http://link.springer.com/article/10.1007/BF00787649

Stephany Watson 2016 The Blood Type Diet" WebMd. N. page web. nov.
08,2017

Stetka, Bret. 2015. "Important Link between the Brain and Immune System
Found," *Scientific American*, July 21.
https://www.scientificamerican.com/article/important-link-between-the-
brain-and-immune-system-found/.

Stockigt, JR and Baverman LE. Update on the Sick Euthyroid
Syndrome. Diseases of the Thyroid. Humana Press, Totowa, NJ, 1997,
pp.49-68

Stress Management Society. 2016. "What Is Stress?" Accessed October 7.
http://www.stress.org.uk/what-is-stress/.

Study.com. 2016. "Macrophages: Definition, Function & Types." Accessed
October 7. http://study.com/ academy/lesson/macrophages-definition-
function-types.html.

Suppversity-Nutrition and exercise science for everyone
(Döhler. 1979; Capen. 1995)
Green tea &your thyroid: Are the T4 & t3 Reducing Effects of 250mg (HED)
Green Tea Catechins Reason For Concern?
http://suppversity.blogspot.ca/2013/03/green-tea-your-thyroid-are-t4-t3.html

The Chalkboard. 2013. "50 Reasons to Drink Wheatgrass Every Day," May 13.
http://thechalkboardmag.com/50-reasons-to-drink-wheatgrass-everyday.

The Free Dictionary, s.v. 2016. "Toxin." Accessed October 7.
http://www.thefreedictionary.com/toxin.

The Gilead Institute of America. 2016. "Your Mind Can Make You Sick."
Accessed October 7. http://www.gilead.net/ health/mindsick.html.

The BMJ "Solanine Poisoning." *British Medical Journal* 2.6203 (1979): 1458–
1459. Print.

The brain from top to bottom. Bruno Dubuc Sept. 2002. N. page. Web Nov.
08,2017

The journal of nutrition 2002http://jn.nutrition.org/content/132/3/329.long

The power of positive thinking: Pathological worry is reduced by thought replacement in Generalized Anxiety Disorder." Web. Oct. 21, 2017

Thomas Rosenthal 2014 "The Little-Known Benefits Of Tocotrienols" Life extension August 2014. N. page. Web. Nov. 08, 2017 Thomson, Helen. 2014. "Human thoughts used to switch on genes," *New Scientist*, November 11. https://www.newscientist.com/article/dn26538-human-thoughts-used-to-switch-on-genes/.

Thompson, Tricia. 2001. "Wheat Starch, Gliadin, and the Gluten-free Diet," *Journal of the Academy of Nutrition and Dietetics* 101(12) 1456-1459. doi: 10.1016/S0002-8223(01)00351-0.

Thyroid Foundation of Canada. 2000. "Thyroid Disorders and Pregnancy." http://www.thyroid.ca/e11a.php.

Thyroid is latest success in regenerative medicine 2016 http://www.nature.com/news/thyroid-is-latest-success- in-regenerative-medicine-1.11574

Thyroid U K better thyroid health "Better thyroid health" http://www.thyroiduk.org.uk/tuk/treatment/fluoride.html Nov. 08, 2017

Tieman, Jill. 2016. "Fructose: How Much Is Safe?" *Real Food Forager*. Accessed October 7. http://realfoodforager.com/ fructose-how-much-is-safe/.

Tom Brimeyer, July 6th, 2015 Hypothyroidism <http://www.forefronthealth.com/overcome-hypothroidism /> web. Oct. 16, 2017

Tommy Jönsson, Stefan Olsson, Bo Ahrén, Thorkild C Bøg-Hansen, Anita Dole and Staffan Lindeberg "Agrarian diet and diseases of affluence – Do evolutionary novel dietary lectins cause leptin resistance?" *BMC Endocrine Disorders*20055:10 \n. page web. nov. 08, 2017

Trans4Mind. 2016. "Acid/Alkaline Balance." Accessed October 7. http://www.trans4mind.com/nutrition/acid-alkaline.html.

(treehugger 2016) http://www.treehugger.com/health/Ancient-heritage-wheat-may-spell-tolerance-for-gluten-sensitive-people.html

Trentini, Dana. 2015. "Cortisol and Thyroid Hormones," *Hypothyroid Mom*, May 8. http://hypothyroidmom.com/cortisol-and-thyroid-hormones/.

—. 2015. "Hashimoto's Disease: The Infection Connection," *Hypothyroid Mom*, April 10. http://hypothyroidmom.com/hashimotos-disease-the-infection-connection/.

Tunsky, Gary. 2016. "pH of the Human Body is Critical for Health," *Health Wealth & Happiness*. Accessed October 7. http://www.relfe.com/health_natural/pH _human_body_balance_health_level_1.html.

Uchigata Y, Spitalnik SL, Tachiwaki O, Salata KF, Notkins AL1987 "Pancreatic islet cell surface glycoproteins containing Gal beta 1-4GlcNAc-R identified by a cytotoxic monoclonal autoantibody." https://www.ncbi.nlm.nih.gov/pmc/articles/PMC2695282/

Udayakumar, Rajangam et al. "Hypoglycaemic and Hypolipidaemic Effects of *Withania Somnifera* Root and Leaf Extracts on Alloxan-Induced Diabetic Rats." *International Journal of Molecular Sciences* 10.5 (2009): 2367–2382. *PMC*. Web. 8 Nov. 2017.

Underground health reporter
An Ancient Herb, Rhodiola Rosea, Increases Mental and Physical Activitieshttp://undergroundhealthreporter.com/rhodiola-rosea-benefits-increase-mental-stamina/

Underground health reporter 2016
http://undergroundhealthreporter.com/apple-cider-vinegar-benefits-home-remedy-for-allergies/

University of Maryland Medical Center. 2016. "Astralagus." Accessed October 7. http://umm.edu/health/medical/ altmed/herb/astragalus.

Urine Therapeutics. 2016. "About Auto Urine Therapy." Accessed October 7. http://www.urinetherapeutics.com/auto_urine_therapy.htm.

—. 2016. "Some Articles on Urine Therapy." Accessed October 7. http://www.urinetherapeutics.com/articles.htm.

Vasconcelos IM, Oliveira JT. "antinutritional properties of plant lectins." 2004 Sep 15;44(4):385-403. NCBI n. page. Web Nov.08,2017

Vanderhaeghe, Lorna. 2016. "Improving Low Thyroid," *Nutritional Ecological Environmental Delivery System*. Accessed October 7. http://www.needs.com/product/HWC08-THY-01/htc_L_Tyrosine.

Victoria M. Indivero Nov. 17, 2015 "Gut bacteria may be to blame for obesity and diabetes" Penn State News web. Oct. 24, 2017

Virginia Hopkins Test Kits. 2016. "How Cortisol Levels Affect Thyroid Function and Aging: Interview with David Zava, Ph.D." Accessed October 7. http://www.virginiahopkinstestkits.com/cortisolzava.html.

W. D. B. Claringbold, J. D. Few & J. H. Renwick "Kinetics and retention of solanidine in man " Journal Xenobiotica Pages 293-302 | Received 27 Nov 1981, Published online: 22 Sep 2008 web. nov. 08,2017

Wadi, Tasaduq. 2014. "Low-Level Autoimmunity," *Professional Education, Testing, and Certification Organization International*. Last modified June 14. http://www.peoi.org/Courses/Coursesen/bioimmune2/temp/ch7a.html.

Walsh, Brian. 2016. "Coffee and Hormones: Here's How Coffee Really Affects Your Health," *Precision Nutrition*. Accessed October 7, 2016

Wang SH, Myc A, Koenig RJ, Bretz JD, Arscott PL, Baker JR. 2000 Jul 25. **"2-** Methoxyestradiol, an endogenous estrogen metabolite, induces thyroid cell apoptosis." National Institute of health. Web. October 15, 2017.

—. 2016. "Green Tea Health Risks: Could Green Tea Actually Be Bad For You?" *Precision Nutrition*. Accessed October 7. http://www.precisionnutrition.com/rr-green-tea-hazards.

Ware, Megan. 2016. "Quinoa: Health Benefits, Nutritional Profile," *Medical News Today*. Last modified July 4. http://www.medicalnewstoday.com/articles/274745.php.

WebMD 2015 10 most-prescribe and top selling medication http://www.webmd.com/news/20150508/most-prescribed-top-selling-drugs

WebMD 2015 most-prescribed-top-selling-drugs http://www.webmd.com/news/20150508/most-prescribed-top-selling-drugs http://www.medscape.com/viewarticle/825053

WebMD. 2016. "Allergies Health Center." Accessed October 7. http://www.webmd.com/allergies/tc/allergic-reaction-topic-overview.

—. 2016. "Causes of Stress." Accessed October 7. http://www.webmd.com/balance/guide/causes-of-stress.

—. 2016. "How Regular Exercise Benefits Teens." Accessed October 7. http://teens.webmd.com/benefits-of-exercise.

WebMD lauric acid 2016 http://www.webmd.com/vitamins-supplements/ingredientmono-1138-lauric%20acid.aspx?activeingredientid=1138&activeingredientname=lauric%20acid

Weiss, Stephen J. 1989. "Tissue Destruction by Neutrophils," *New England Journal of Medicine* 1989 (320) 365-376. doi: 10.1056/NEJM198902093200606.

Wentz, Izabella. 2016. "Is It Possible To Recover Thyroid Function In Hashimoto's?" *Thyroid Pharmacist.* Accessed October 7. http://thyroidpharmacist.com/articles/is-it-possible-to-recover-thyroid-function-in-hashimotos.

White, MV. 1990." The Role of Histamine in Allergic Diseases," *Journal of Allergy and Clinical Immunology* 86(4 Pt 2):599-605. https://www.ncbi.nlm.nih.gov/pubmed/1699987.

Wikipedia, s.v. 2016. "Alcohol and Cortisol." Accessed October 7. https://en.wikipedia.org/wiki/Alcohol_and_cortisol.

—. 2016. "Allergy." Accessed October 7. https://en.wikipedia.org/ wiki/Allergy.

—. 2016. "Anti-Thyroid Antibodies." Accessed October 7. https://en.wikipedia.org/wiki/Anti-thyroid_autoantibodies.

—. 2016. "Anti-Transglutaminase Antibodies." Accessed October 7. https://en.wikipedia.org/wiki/Anti-transglutaminase_antibodies.

—. 2016. "Autoimmunity." Accessed October 7. https://en.wikipedia. org/wiki/Autoimmunity.

—. 2016. "Cortisol." Accessed October 7. https://en.wikipedia.org/ wiki/Cortisol.

—. 2016. "Essential Amino Acid." Accessed October 7. https://en.wikipedia.org/wiki/Essential_amino_acid.

—. 2016. "Galactose." Accessed October 7. https://en.wikipedia.org/ wiki/Galactose.

—. 2016. "Immunity (Medical)." Accessed October 7. https://en.wiki pedia.org/wiki/Immunity_(medical).

—. 2016. "Inflammation." Accessed October 7. https://en.wikipedia. org/wiki/Inflammation.

—. 2016. "Major Histocompatibility Complex." Accessed October 7. https://en.wikipedia.org/wiki/Major_histocompatibility_complex.

—. 2016. "Miracle." Accessed October 7. https://en.wikipedia.org/ wiki/Miracle.

—. 2016. "Neurotransmitter." Accessed October 7. https://en.wiki pedia.org/wiki/Neurotransmitter.

—. 2016. "Postpartum Thyroiditis." Accessed October 7. https://en.wikipedia.org/wiki/Postpartum_thyroiditis.

—. 2016. "Stress (Biology)." Accessed October 7. https://en.wikipedia.org/wiki/Stress_(biology).

—. 2016. "Thyrotropin Receptor." Accessed October 7. https://en.wikipedia.org/wiki/Thyrotropin_receptor.

—. 2016. "Urine therapy." Accessed October 7. https://en.wikipedia.org/wiki/Urine_therapy.

Wiley Online Library
Thyroid and pituitary hormones in relation to regeneration. 1. The effect of anterior pituitary hormone on regeneration of the hind leg in normal and thyroidectomized newts.
http://onlinelibrary.wiley.com/doi/10.1002/jez.1400830307/abstract

Wood-Moen, Robin. 2011. "Herbs to Avoid With Hypothyroidism," *LIVESTRONG*, May 11. http://www.livestrong.com/article/440613-herbs-to-avoid-with-hypothyroidism/.

The World's Healthiest Foods. 2016. "Flaxseeds." Accessed October 7. http://www.whfoods.com/ genpage.php?tname=foodspice&dbid=81.

World healthies food 2016. "Ginger." Accessed October 7. http://www.whfoods.com/ genpage.php?tname=foodspice&dbid=72.

—. 2016. "Ginger." Accessed October 7. http://www.whfoods.com/ genpage.php?tname=foodspice&dbid=72.

Yamamoto F, Cid E, Yamamoto M, Blancher A. "ABO research in the modern era of genomics." 2012 Apr;26(2):103-18. doi: 10.1016/j.tmrv.2011.08.002. Epub 2011 Sep 23. NCBI n. page. Web. Nov. 08,2017

Yang F, Basu TK, Ooraikul B "Studies on germination conditions and antioxidant contents of wheat grain." 2001 Jul;52(4):319-30. NCBI n. page. Web Nov, 08, 2017

Yevdokimova NY and Yefimov AS. "Effects of wheat germ agglutinin and concanavalin A on the accumulation of glycosaminoglycans in pericellular matrix of human dermal fibroblasts. A comparison with insilin" 2001;48(2):563-72.NCBI n. page web. Nov. 08, 2017

Yin J, Xing H and Ye J. 2008 "Efficacy of berberine in patients with type 2 diabetes mellitus." 2008 May;57(5):712-7. doi: 10.1016/j.metabol.2008.01.013. NCBI web Nov. 08, 2017

Zouali, Moncef. 2015. "Natural Antibodies," *eLS*. John Wiley & Sons Ltd, Chichester. doi: 10.1002/9780470015902.a0001213.pub3.

AUTHOR PAGE

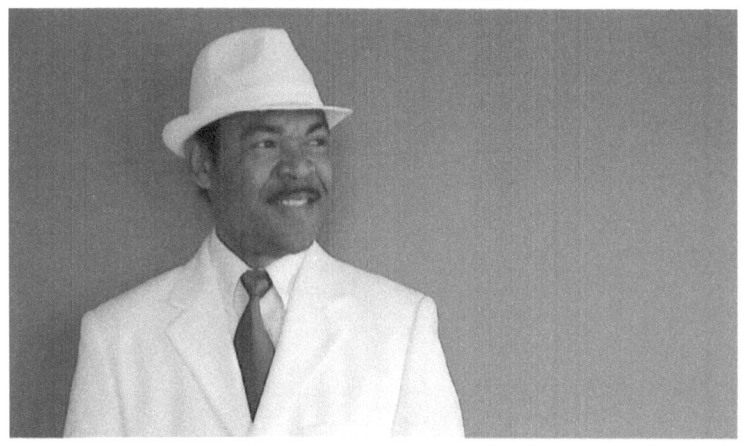

Irvin Symonette was born June 07, 1960 in the gold-mining village of Siuna, on the north-eastern shores of Nicaragua. He left his homeland in 1983 due to political instability. In 1985 he found refuge in Canada where he found and married his missing half: Carol Wilson. Their union produced four children: one beauty, Gita and three beasts: Remo, Niko and Nea.

He is an entrepreneur, motivational speaker and an avid scholar of Biblical principles for success. The onset of Hashimoto thyroiditis in 2010, led him on a 5-year journey, where he discovered one profound truth: Hashimoto autoimmune disease is not the end. Everyone can experience remission just by following a few basic health principles.